# ASPERGER'S

# SYNDROME

# TABLE OF CONTENTS

# INTRODUCTION

Asperger syndrome (AS), also referred to as Asperger's, is a developmental disorder characterized by deficiencies in social and communication skills. The exact cause of Asperger's is unknown and the prevalence is not firmly established, due partly to the use of different sets of diagnostic criteria.

Asperger's is often not identified in early childhood, and many individuals do not receive a diagnosis until after puberty or when they are adults. Teens with Asperger's are usually aware of their differences and recognize when they need support from family. There are instances where teens do not know they have Asperger's personalities until they are having difficulties with relationships in adult life.

Asperger's is a condition in which there is:

1. Impairment in social interaction

2. The presence of restricted, repetitive and

stereotyped behaviors and interests

3. Significant impairment in important areas of functioning

4. No significant delay in language

5. No significant delay in cognitive development, self-help skills, or adaptive behaviors (other than social interaction)

6. The symptoms must not be better accounted for by another specific pervasive developmental disorder or schizophrenia

Asperger's is characterized by:

1. Limited interests or preoccupation with a subject to the exclusion of other activities

2. Repetitive behaviors or rituals

3. Peculiarities in speech and language

4. Socially and emotionally inappropriate behavior and interpersonal interaction

5. Problems with nonverbal communication

## 6. Clumsy and uncoordinated motor movements

Most adolescents with moderate to severe Asperger's will show little or no interest in others. They may seem to be totally unaware of their peers' presence, or they may appear indifferent when peers try to interact.

Some youngsters with Asperger's get very nervous just with the thought of approaching others and may choose to avoid it at all costs. Their avoidance may appear as if they are not interested in others.

Yet some adolescents with Asperger's will not avoid interacting with others. They are eager to communicate, though, often in a clumsy, in-your-face way.

Children with Asperger's are often the target of bullying at school due to their "strange" behavior, language, interests, and impaired ability to interact in socially expected ways to nonverbal cues, particularly in interpersonal conflict. Children with Asperger's may be extremely literal and may have difficulty interpreting and responding to sarcasm or banter.

Most children with Asperger's want to be social, but fail to socialize successfully, which can lead to later withdrawal and social behavior, especially in adolescence. Teens with Asperger's often get along a lot better with those considerably older or younger than them, rather than those their own age.

A child with Asperger's might be regarded by teachers as a "problem child" or a "poor performer." The child's extremely low tolerance for "ordinary" and "mediocre" tasks (e.g., homework) can easily become frustrating. A teacher may consider the child arrogant, spiteful, and insubordinate. This misunderstanding, in combination with the child's anxieties, can result in problematic behavior (e.g., violent and angry outbursts, withdrawal).

Although there is no single feature that all teens with Asperger's share, difficulties with social behavior are nearly universal and are one of the most important defining criteria.

Teens with Asperger's have difficulty empathizing with others (i.e., putting themselves in someone else's shoes), and may lack the ability to communicate their own emotional state, resulting in well-meaning remarks that may offend, or finding it hard to know what is "acceptable".

Teens with Asperger's may have trouble understanding the emotions of other people (e.g., messages conveyed by facial expression, eye contact, and body language). Thus, teens with Asperger's might be seen as egotistical, selfish or uncaring. In most cases, these are unfair labels because they are neurologically unable to understand other people's emotional states. They are usually surprised, upset or remorseful when told that their actions are hurtful or inappropriate.

Individuals with Asperger's do not lack emotions. However, the concrete nature of emotional attachments they have (i.e., to objects rather than to people) often seems curious or can even be a cause of concern to people who do not share their perspective.

Teens with Asperger's may have little patience for things outside their narrow interests. In school, they may be perceived as highly intelligent underachievers or overachievers, clearly capable of outperforming their peers in their field of interest, yet persistently unmotivated to do regular homework assignments.

Some children with Asperger's experience varying degrees of sensory overload and are extremely sensitive to touch, smells, sounds, tastes, and sights.

Sensory overload may exacerbate problems faced by such children at school, where levels of noise in the classroom can become intolerable for them. A child with Asperger's can become distracted, agitated, or even aggressive if unwanted touch, sounds, smells, etc. persist.

Treatment for Asperger's consists of therapies that apply behavior management strategies and address poor communication skills, obsessive or repetitive routines, and physical clumsiness.

Currently, the most effective treatment involves a combination of psychotherapy, special education, behavior modification, and support for families. Some children with Asperger's Disorder will also benefit from medication.

A typical treatment program generally includes:

1. Social skills training, to teach the skills to more successfully interact with others

2. Cognitive behavioral therapy to help in better managing emotions that may be explosive or anxious, and to cut back on obsessive interests and repetitive routines

3. Medication for co-existing conditions such as depression and anxiety

4. Occupational or physical therapy to assist with poor motor coordination

5. Speech therapy to help with the trouble of the "give and take" in normal conversation

6. Parent training and support, to teach parents behavioral techniques to use at home.

All these treatments will be treated in details in this book.

Children with Asperger's can learn to manage their differences, but they may continue to find social situations and personal relationships challenging.

Many adults with Asperger's are able to work successfully in mainstream jobs, although they may continue to need encouragement and moral support to maintain an independent life.

Teens with Asperger's report a feeling of being unwillingly detached from the world around them. As an adult, they may have difficulty getting married due to poor social skills.

On the other hand, some adults with Asperger's do get married, get graduate degrees, become wealthy, and hold jobs. The intense focus and tendency to work things out logically often grant those people with Asperger's a high level of ability in their field of interest.

When these special interests coincide with a materially or socially useful task, the person with Asperger's often can lead a profitable life. For example, the child obsessed with a particular computer game may grow up to be an accomplished computer programmer.

The outcome for children with Asperger's Disorder is generally more promising than for those with autism. Due to their higher level of intellectual functioning, many of these children successfully finish high school and attend college. Although problems with social interaction and awareness persist, they can also develop lasting relationships with family and friends.

Let's get started.

# CHAPTER ONE
# WHAT IS ASPERGER'S SYNDROME?

Asperger's syndrome is a developmental disorder related to the autistic spectrum but at a much higher level of functioning. Unlike those with autism, those who have Asperger's syndrome generally learn the same way average people do, learning to speak at a young age and eventually attending school in the same classes and at the same age of their peers. Like autism, however, those with Asperger's syndrome may have trouble understanding social or communication skills. This often results in being viewed as 'weird' by those around them who aren't familiar with the disorder.

Asperger's syndrome is typically diagnosed at an early age, but because those who have it are on the higher functioning end of the autism scale, it can go undiagnosed well into adulthood. This has been especially common in the past when the disorder wasn't as well known and understood as it has become in recent years. Similar to autism, there is no cure and the exact cause of the disorder is unknown, however, it is possible to manage the symptoms, including clumsiness, obsessive routines, and sensitivity to environmental changes. This is done with behavioral therapy, resulting in many adults with Asperger's syndrome appearing mostly 'normal' with the exception of lack of social skills.

The lack of social skills doesn't mean that all adults with Asperger's appear rude, but rather they have trouble understanding social cues. For example, it's not uncommon for those with Asperger's syndrome to share a deep passion for something, whether it be horses or molecules. They may want to talk about this passion constantly, despite the listener growing visibly annoyed. This is because they don't understand that sighing or looking at a watch means the listener is uninterested.

Due to this extreme passion, many adults with Asperger's syndrome end up excelling in careers involving their interest. It's not uncommon for adults with Asperger's to become CEO's or other high ranking positions because unlike other employees, they don't spend their time socializing with others, but rather learning as much as humanly possible about their passion.

What is the Asperger Syndrome diagnostic scale?

The Asperger Syndrome Diagnostic Scale, also known as ASDS, is a tool used to screen for children who might meet criteria for Asperger's Syndrome. This quickly administered standardized test only takes approximately 15 minutes to complete. It is appropriate for children ages five through

18 years old.

The screening tool is standardized and uses percentiles to give an AS Quotient. This score predicts the likelihood that a child or adolescent has Asperger's Syndrome. The test covers behaviors across several domains, including cognitive, maladaptive, social, sensory, motor, and language.

The behaviors addressed are those behaviors typically seen in children with Asperger's, as well as behaviors that are seen in children without an Autistic Disorder.

The Asperger Syndrome Diagnostic Scale has an administrative qualification level of B. This means that individuals who administer the ASDS must have a degree from an accredited four-year college. This degree must be completed in psychology, counseling, or speech and language pathology. The individual must also have completed coursework in test interpretation, psychometrics, educational statistics, or measurement theory or a license indicating appropriate training in the ethics and competency required for using psychological tests.

The respondent for the ASDS can be one of several individuals who are very familiar with the child or adolescent being tested. Parents and siblings are often the primary respondents.

The child's service providers, such as speech and language pathologists, therapists, and teachers can also act as respondents.

The Asperger Syndrome Diagnostic Scale cannot be used in isolation to provide a diagnosis of Asperger's. The ASDS is a screening tool to indicate the likelihood of the individual having Asperger's. The AS Quotient can be used to indicate whether a professional should further evaluate the child in order to receive an official formal diagnosis.

One concern with the ASDS is that it has not been shown to reliably differentiate between Asperger Syndrome and the other subtypes of Autism Spectrum Disorder. Since the symptoms of Asperger are also similar to the symptoms of PDD-NOS and Autistic Disorder, a qualified team of autism professionals must do further evaluation. This can help determine what subset of Autism Spectrum Disorder the individual has.

A benefit of the ASDS is that it not only provides an overall AS Quotient, but it also gives scores for each of the individual domains on the test. The individual results in the cognitive, language, social, maladaptive, and sensor motor subscales can assist the professional in determining specific areas of deficit and difficulty in the child. These scores can be especially helpful in treatment planning and determining areas for further testing.

The results of the ADSD also have other non-clinical purposes. They can also be used to help draft goals for the child's IEP or school intervention plan. The test can also be given annually as a way to measure growth and progress across the different domains in an individual already diagnosed with Asperger Syndrome.

What types of Asperger's tests are available for adults?

Like previously stated, Asperger syndrome is a pervasive developmental disorder characterized by significant impairments in social interaction and stereotyped patterns of behavior. What distinguishes Asperger Syndrome from other Autism Spectrum Disorders is the lack of any significant delay in language or cognitive ability. Asperger Syndrome is not as easy to diagnose as other disorders of the Autism Spectrum, so it is quite common for a person with Asperger to receive the diagnosis as an adult, even though the problems began in childhood. There are several tests and assessments that are designed to determine whether an adult has Asperger Syndrome or one of the other Autism Spectrum Disorders.

The ADI (Autism Diagnostic Interview-Revised) is an interview-based assessment that is used to ask questions of a parent, or if the parent is not available, some other person who knew the individual as a child. The questions are designed to determine whether the adult had problems with social interactions as a child and to rule out other forms of autism. The ADI is effective, but it is limited since the parent may no longer be available, and it takes about three hours to administer.

The AQ (Autism Spectrum Quotient) is a much shorter screening device used to identify adults who may have Asperger Syndrome or Autism. This instrument contains 50 questions that relate to the areas of social skill, attention switching, attention to detail, communication and imagination. The subject responds to each question with "definitely agree," "slightly agree," "slightly disagree" and "definitely disagree." The responses to these questions show the degree to which the subject has features typical of people with Autism or Asperger Syndrome.

Another Asperger screening instrument is the EQ (Empathy Quotient), a 15 item questionnaire used to determine the degree to which an individual cannot understand the feelings and thoughts of others. Though this is a really short assessment that focuses on only one area of development, it has a very strong correlation with the presence of Asperger Syndrome.

Where does Asperger's come from?

So where does Asperger's comes from?

Before I tell you, allow me to describe a quality which underlies the whole of Emergence Personality Theory. This quality? Blamelessness; the idea that no one consciously causes their pain. This includes the parents of kids with Asperger's. Not one of them ever causes their child to get Asperger's.

Where does it come from then? It was once normal for all of us to focus on sensation at the expense of our social relationships. When? In the first six months of life. Unfortunately, some babies never expand beyond this focus. Thus, they incur the condition we call, Kanner's Autism. In the second six months of life, we all have another norm. We focus on learning how to use the ability we mastered in our first six months; sensation itself, to sense the things in our environment. Here again, some few babies unfortunately never focus beyond this point. In their case, we call what they have, OCPD; Obsessive Compulsive

Personality Disorder. The compulsion to sense the things in their environment at the expense of connecting to people.

And Asperger's then? Asperger's comes into being sometime during a baby's second year of life. How? Well, consider what is normal for babies to focus on during this stage in their lives. They focus on learning to understand the things they've learned to sense in the prior stage of their development. Thus, if babies do not move past this focus, they remain intensely interested in learning for learning's sake, even to the point wherein they never learn to connect to people.

Is there a fourth norm then? Absolutely. From age two to age four, kids normally rebel against any pressure put on them to simply parrot what other folks have learned. The "terrible two's," remember? So what does this turn out to be if the baby never loses this focus? ADD. Attention Deficit Disorder. And yes, I know medically minded folks now call this condition, ADHD. However, it seems incredibly silly to diagnose a kid as having ADHD without HD. Which happens to be the most common version of this lab rat label.

What could we be doing to better help these folks?

So what could we be doing to better help these folks? Well, in the case of Asperger's, we could be focusing our efforts on getting these folks to make "connecting" more important than "information." Note, I haven't simply said, teach them better social skills.

In truth, teaching mouth readers to read eyes is a lot easier than you might imagine. In fact, given they believe you have something valid to say, folks with Asperger's are among the best folks of all to teach.

What else could we be doing? We could stop telling them they have a disease. They do not. They have a style of relating to the world which was once normal for all of us but no longer is.

During this time, we all made learning the meaning of things our special interest. Moreover, in babies aged one to two, this focus is absolutely normal. In people with Asperger's, however, this tendency never leaves them. Thus, what was once normal now impairs their very ability to see the beauty in people. And renders them unable to do much more than parrot authentic social connections. The very thing that ADD kids hate doing. Which in part explains why AS kids have the most difficult time with ADD kids.

What else could we be doing to help? For one thing, we could pay more attention to the way "focusing on information more than people" plays out in the very nature of peoples' language skills.

"Fuzzy" and "fussy." Two very different qualities. Especially when applied to language. The ability to help here would come from teaching both those with Asperger's and those who do not have it, to speak to each other in the other's language. In effect, they both become bilingual, in that they both learn to speak "fussy" and they both learn to speak "fussy." Learning this alone has changed the whole outlook on the world.

As well as allowing them to socially connect to others for the first time in their life.

One more thing we could be doing is we could stop reminding people with Asperger's that some few folks with Asperger's became world changers. Why stop saying this? Because this only makes them feel even more inept. And more like failures.

People with Asperger's are not failures. They are simply in the minority, both language wise and interest wise. Moreover, to see this as true, simply imagine our world were it not for people like them. Easier in some ways. Yes. Certainly. But without the special interests of those few who have changed the world?

# CHAPTER TWO

# HOW TO IDENTIFY ATYPICAL ASPERGERS SYNDROME?

The incidence of Asperger's Syndrome is on the rise. Asperger's is one of the Autistic Spectrum Disorders, or ASD's. Whenever we see a spike in the incidence of a disorder, I always ask the questions "is this disorder/syndrome occurring more frequently? Or, are we simply diagnosing it more often? Is it the new 'fashionable' diagnosis?" These are important professional questions. Labels and diagnoses can shape a future for the better or worse. We shouldn't diagnose lightly. Many implications follow a diagnosis.

I am seeing with more frequency, elements of Asperger's Syndrome in children but an absence of some key identifying symptoms. The diagnostic criteria listed in the Diagnostic and Statistical Manual IV (DSM-IV, the manual authorized by the American

Psychiatric Association) is far too long to reprint here in a book. Some highlights are as follows:

1. Qualitative impairment in social interaction.

2. Restricted repetitive and stereotyped patterns of behavior, interests, and activities.

3. The disturbance causes clinically significant impairment in social, occupational, or other important areas of functioning.

4. There is no significant general delay in language (e.g., single words used by age 2 years, communicative phrases used by age 3 years).

5. There is no clinically significant delay in the cognitive development of age-appropriate self-help skills, adaptive behavior (other than in social interaction), and curiosity about the environment in

childhood.

6. Criteria are not met for another specific Pervasive Developmental Disorder or Schizophrenia.

I am using the term in this chapter "Atypical Asperger's Syndrome" to refer to children who seem to meet some of the criteria but not all. Things just don't seem to click for these kids. They just don't engage the way other children do.

Atypical Aspergers may be best discussed by comparing it to some other possible diagnoses that we may be ruled out. They are as follows:

1. Social Anxiety Disorder: Children with this disorder may appear quite shy. They are hesitant to engage with other children. They prefer the company of adults. In differentiating this from Atypical Asperger's, the Asperger's child isn't remotely upset, concerned or bothered by the fact that they

aren't included in the group. Or, they are included in the group but remain somewhat permanently distant. They can play side by side with other children without really interacting with the other child.

2. Low Intellectual Functioning: Upon initial observation, the Atypical Aspergers child may appear dull or lacking in intelligence. The low intellectual functioning child generally will perform poorly in school and require basic skills level classes.

The Atypical Asperger's child, however, is most often bright. They do well on test despite appearing lost or disinterested.

Asperger's Syndrome children typically make poor eye contact, speak in limited phrases, are tangential, prefer social isolation. They display a lack of spontaneous seeking to share enjoyment, interests or achievements with others. They also display a lack of social or emotional reciprocity.

I am seeing Atypical Asperger's children who make good eye contact. They are often capable of conducting a conversation. Parents and teachers report that these children are less skilled in conversation with their peer age group. They may spontaneously share experiences or achievements but often at inappropriate times, interjecting such as a discussion somewhat randomly. And although they are bright, if I were their age I wouldn't be very interested in what they talk about. They appear immature because they are socially immature.

For some reason, the Atypical Asperger's child doesn't seem interested in athletics and also not very good at them. I don't fully understand the neurology involved but I'm suspecting a connection.

Fashionable Syndrome?

I was discussing Asperger's with my friend just last week. We were looking at the homes of America's richest tech guys, Bill Gates, Steve Jobs and "the facebook guy" Mark Zuckerberg. Our conversation led us to "how many of these very bright and creative guys have Asperger's." And we must make an important point, just because someone appears socially awkward doesn't mean that they have any disorder at all, let alone Aspergers. It was simply a conversation. I am not diagnosing any of these individuals from afar and have no idea if any of them have any version of Asperger's Syndrome. The point though is that he told me that in his 20 something age group it has become "fashionable" to say that you have Asperger's.

It is sort of a badge of honor and an easy explanation for ones "quirkiness" now in social situations. Guys in bars and clubs are using this to create an aura of "intellectual elite" associated with themselves. I see it as a way of saying "I'm really better and smarter than you and you couldn't possibly really understand me so don't even try." It's the new "I'm a nerd" declaration. Remember when being called a nerd was an insult? Remember when it became a badge of honor years later? This also points out that the more evident cases of adult Atypical Asperger's Syndrome occur in bright creative people. I don't believe that the incidence is higher in bright people than less bright people. We simply notice it more because we notice high achievers overall more than lesser achievers.

This may seem strange or unusual at first glance. But think of how often you hear people referring to "my ADD." I hear this all the time. It's become an excuse for everything. Any time someone forgets fails to complete a project or return a phone call promptly, they announce that it's there ADD.

So to think that now the fashionable disorder or "disorder du jour" is something called Asperger's doesn't surprise me in the least.

We, as a society, are influenced by media and current fashion. All of the Autistic Spectrum disorders are in "fashion" in the media.

And this points to concern. Certain diagnoses become popular. Think of this timeline. The popular diagnosis in the 1980s was "Chronic Fatigue Syndrome." I bet you forgot about that one. When was the last time you heard of someone having it? Not recently, eh. Where did it go? What was the cure? In the 1990's ADD and ADHD came into full bloom, even though we were talking about it in the '80s. They've hung on pretty well too. But in the 2000's we began to see a lot of children with Bipolar Disorder.

We all function within a range on a scale. Atypical Asperger's is simply on a different part of that scale than most people are accustomed.

Here are some basic considerations if you question whether your child may have a form of Asperger's Syndrome:

Your child is bright but doesn't interact well with peers.

Your child doesn't have a normal filter when expressing himself. He says inappropriate things at inappropriate times.

He doesn't seem too bothered to be on the "outside" of things socially.

He is preoccupied or his focus on certain activities is abnormal or unusually intense.

He is preoccupied with parts of objects in a way that others are not.

His conversation runs to things that are completely dis-interesting to others, and he fails to notice.

This is not an exhaustive or comprehensive

list. But it's a good start. Get a comprehensive assessment if you think this may be a problem.

## SIGNS AND SYMPTOMS OF ASPERGER'S

Asperger's syndrome is considered as one of the pervasive developmental disorders and with the main signs and symptoms of Asperger's centering on the impairment of social and communicative abilities. Current statistics suggest that up to 3 out of every 10,000 children will be diagnosed with Asperger's syndrome and boys are 3 or 4 times more likely to suffer from the disorder than girls.

Here is a list of the most common signs and symptoms associated with Asperger's syndrome, but please bear in mind that every child's case of Asperger's is different and just because a majority of kids showed one symptom, doesn't mean every child has or will.

1. As stated above, a majority, but not all, of Asperger's syndrome symptoms, are social in nature. The first symptom that many parents or teachers notice in a child that has Asperger's is a lack of understanding of social cues or the inability to understand body language. This can extend to the basic ability to start and end a conversation as well as the idea of waiting to speak until the person you are speaking to has finished.

2. Most children that show signs of Asperger's syndrome do not like any change in their routine. This is also a common symptom of the classic form of autism, as well.

3. A common symptom that is almost always associated with Asperger's syndrome is the apparent lack of empathy. Empathy, or the ability to sense the emotions and emotional state of another person, is part of an Asperger's patient social failings. It is easy to see how a lack of

empathy can make even the simplest social interaction extremely awkward.

4. An Asperger's child may not be able to understand the subtle differences in tone and meaning during social interaction. It makes things like understanding humor or plays-on-words like puns almost impossible to understand. Also, things like sarcasm tend to be extremely difficult for an Asperger's child to understand.

The child may also not use the proper speech patterns and not vary their tone of speech much or at all. Again, this only adds to the social awkwardness of a child with this disorder.

5. Adding to the already overwhelming social awkwardness is the fact that many Asperger's sufferers will tend to use much more formal or advanced language for their age. While it might seem cute and even endearing when conversing with adults, with other children it can be extremely

alienating.

6. A child with Asperger's syndrome also tends to avoid eye contact when speaking to you. They either look at the ground or just look away from the person to whom they are speaking.

7. Despite these socially awkward traits, many Asperger's children will be quite talkative, usually about one topic that they may seem to be obsessed with. It can be something as simple as baseball stats or something obscure that they just saw on television.

8. They may also have an unusual posture or walking style and move in a clumsy manner.

While Asperger's syndrome doesn't present the serious problems that classic autism does, it can still be a very tough disorder to deal with. With the proper assistance, however, a child diagnosed with Asperger's can live a happy and full life.

# CHAPTER THREE
# ASPERGERS SYNDROME
# BEHAVIORAL ASPECT

It is unknown as to what causes Asperger's syndrome. The behavioral aspect of this disorder can render children with Aspergers to behave ⏹uite strangely and at times they can even unintentionally make remarks that can be quite rude and painful towards others while being so unaware of their effect from the remarks. This is usually a result of the social disconnect found within children showing signs of Aspergers as well as their lack of imagination that can make it quite easy not to show empathy towards their peers.

Many children with Aspergers grow up to become teens not interested in the latest fads, social norms or conventional ways of thinking. Normally children with Aspergers Syndrome deem themselves to being creative and original thinkers in pursuit of their own goals and interests. Sometimes Aspergers teens can excel in class due to their strong preferences for rules and structure.

Teens with Aspergers can excel in certain fields due to their narrow focus of interest. For example, a teen with Asperger's syndrome may excel greatly in math due to their narrow interest in the subject but struggle in English or History class due to their high disinterest in the field brought on by the sole preoccupation to only be interested in Math.

Parents should be encouraging towards children and teens with Aspergers. Teachers should learn how to respond to students with Asperger's syndrome, but patience is a virtue when dealing with the signs of Asperger's syndrome in children, teens or adults. Every child is different and it is important to establish a safe and trusting environment that can enable the child to reach out if help is sought. Good communication skills can only be learned if the child with Asperger's syndrome feels that they are in a safe and welcoming environment.

.

## MANAGING ASPERGERS SYNDROME BEHAVIOR

For many, the proper diagnosis of Aspergers Syndrome may give rise to the larger problem of how to manage Asperger's syndrome behavior. There are guidelines which can be of assistance in establishing practices designed to help those with Aspergers syndrome develop skills which can lessen the impact of the disorder. These include the following:

Teaching basic skills and concepts should be undertaken with sufferers of Aspergers syndrome in an explicit and deliberate manner with an explanation as to how the parts fit into a larger whole.

Social awareness may need to be instructively promoted rather than intuitively learned, with the focus being given to specific examples of appropriate behavior in discreet situations. A clear emphasis on the difference between the perceptions of a person with Aspergers syndrome as distinct from others should be explained.

Regular visitation of problem-solving techniques, with a focus on providing step-by-step strategies to effectively recognize and deal with common everyday difficulties.

The practice of simultaneously interpreting visual and auditory stimuli should be cultivated with a view to assisting an Aspergers syndrome sufferer in classifying non-verbal behavior, and understanding how that behavior correlates with verbal communication. The implications of eye-contact, non-verbal communication such as hand gestures, facial expression, and obvious body language should be explored. Changes in tone, inflection, and figurative language should be instructed broadly, with increasing specificity over time.

Self-sufficiency may be enhanced by increasing the adaptive skills of those with Aspergers syndrome. Rote learning of specific activities, such as travel or meeting strangers, should be verbally instructed and rehearsed in order that sequential repetition can give rise to learned behavior.

Subsequent reinforcement of those routines should be undertaken by coordination and communication with those responsible for the individual's ongoing care, welfare, and development. Consistency in routine will be a significant factor in its assimilation by the individual into behavior patterns.

Self-awareness and evaluation may need to

be independently encouraged to both enable individuals with Aspergers syndrome to perceive appropriate behavior in different social circumstances and to assist with self-esteem when such situations are successfully managed. Again, pre-learned strategies applied in practice to specific examples will compliment the cognitive abilities of those with Aspergers.

The establishment of a 'safety-net' for circumstances where an Aspergers syndrome individual encounters a novel situation should be implemented, with a pre-planned course of action to be undertaken.

The link between certain anxiety provoking experiences and resulting feelings of frustration and depression should be explicitly taught in a 'cause and effect' manner in order to engender within the Aspergers syndrome individual some insight into their own emotions. This can also assist in gaining empathetic response by enabling the individual to have some awareness of the feelings of others. The individual with Aspergers syndrome should be encouraged to monitor their own speech patterns, and be instructed as to the interpretation which others may place upon it.

To assist with age-appropriate communication with their peer group, Aspergers syndrome individuals may be assisted by instructions on how to manage topics of discussion, the importance of topic expansion, closing discussions, and gaining comfort in mutual engagement.

Ultimately, a combination of learned behavior may be explored to establish guidelines to prevent disruptive behavior, assist in more intuitive decision making, and participate in open forms of communication.

The integration of these types of behavior

management strategies can be assisted by their coordination both in the home and in the case of children, at school. With proper management and professional assistance, a pro-active and integrated approach to managing Aspergers syndrome behavior can be of both short term and long term benefits to those afflicted by it.

## HOW TO COPE ASPERGERS SYNDROME SYMPTOMS?

As many children with autism and other developmental delay disorders, Aspergers syndrome symptoms include having difficulties with social interactions. Children with Aspergers syndrome symptoms usually have the most problems when it comes to the interpretation of nonverbal cues given by other people such as body language and facial expressions.

Forming friendships with other peers can be a difficult task because Aspergers symptoms make it difficult for normal social interactions to take place.

Many people with Aspergers syndrome symptoms have a low desire to share their experiences or interests with other people, for example, if a child with Aspergers syndrome builds a toy, they are more likely to keep the discovery to themselves than to share and brag about it to others such as most children do.

Children with Aspergers have an impressive vocabulary with the exception of course of social skills lacking. Being obsessively interested in a single particular object or subject is yet another defining characteristic of Aspergers syndrome symptoms.

A child with Aspergers syndrome symptoms may choose to become fixated on one single particular subject and be neglectful in taking interest in much else. They can obsessively seek to find advanced information about clocks, maps, and other single topics, but may become quite inflexible even rigid in their habits, routines and rituals.

Odd mannerisms can also arise from children with Aspergers. Hand flapping, as well as other postures, may contribute to making a child with Aspergers to appear clumsy. While growing up, children exhibiting Aspergers symptoms may grow up being seen as "odd", even "eccentric" later on as adults.

Anxiety can at times arise in the case of social interactions, especially in fairly new social situations. Children with Aspergers symptoms can at times have debilitating compulsions due to the introduction of new social situations. There is medical treatment available for anxiety, however, parents, as well as educational facilities, are encouraged to remain patient and to continue the needed social skills training.

## ASPERGERS SYMPTOMS ARE TREATABLE

Aspergers is a disorder that is very hard to diagnose because it has variable symptoms and no two people with this disorder act the same. To realize if your child has Aspergers is not an easy thing. However, there are some symptoms you can try to observe. Asperger's treatment is only possible by managing the symptoms and because the symptoms are varied, every child with Aspergers must be treated according to their own symptoms.

Children with Aspergers have normal cognitive and language development. The problems start when they interact with other children. People with Aspergers Syndrome have difficulties understanding the facial expressions of the others, they don't like eye contact and they don't understand metaphoric statements. They show no physical signs like children with Down syndrome.

Also, no genetic reason or chemical imbalance is found for Aspergers Syndrome. This disorder is considered to be in autism spectrum. This means that it is a kind of autism, differentiating only by its severity or rather its lack of severity. Aspergers is on the high functioning end of autism spectrum. It has very similar characteristics like eye contact problem or repetitive behavior but these symptoms are less severe in children with Asperger's disorder.

There are extensive tests to be able to diagnose Aspergers Syndrome. Once these tests are conducted and a diagnosis is reached, it is very essential to let the child know about the disorder. Children with this disorder see the world from a different window. They are very capable to understand the behaviors of their peers.

Because of their disorder, they are generally isolated and they don't like to be around people. However, this does not mean that they don't like people or they don't want to have friends.

They like people and they would like to have friends but they can't show their feelings and their facial expression usually make people think otherwise. They are extremely intelligent and have a tendency to learn excessive information about a single subject.

When children with this disorder grow up, they usually become very successful people in the areas they choose. The hardest time they live in their childhood and adolescence. To give them the highest possible quality of life their parents must undertake the hard job of protecting them.

Aspergers is a difficult disorder to deal with. However if we compare it to other disorders like Dawn or autistic disorder, the people with Aspergers are luckier. They can have a full, productive life. They can get married, have children and work in a normal environment.

When it is diagnosed early, Asperger's treatment shows more promise. Some symptoms can be alleviated more easily when they don't turn into bad habits. Once the person with Aspergers understands the differences with other people and problems he can face everything becomes easier.

# CHAPTER FOUR
# ASPERGER SYNDROME IN ADULTS

Asperger syndrome in adults may be hard for the sufferers and can be a challenge for the people around them as well. Although there is no total cure for this disorder, you can help them cope up with this developmental disorder and live at least a normal life.

Although different persons can exhibit different symptoms, there are signs that are common among sufferers. The most common are difficulty in social interaction and communication and the difficulty to understand body language.

Other signs and symptoms of Asperger syndrome in adults may include their difficulty in abstract thinking, difficulty in empathizing with others, difficulty in understanding other nonverbal communication such as facial expressions, eye contact, and body language. Sufferers of Asperger's syndrome can often be misinterpreted as rude, disrespectful or selfish as they may not be capable of understanding the feelings of the people around them. They may also find it difficult to see a situation in another person's point of view and may not be able to understand appropriate social behavior.

Understand also that people with Asperger syndrome may find it hard to control their emotions and feelings such as anger, anxiety, and depression. Thus, if you are dealing with adults having this disorder, or you may be in a relationship with a person having this disorder, it is best to have tons of patience and understanding and teach them to cope up with such symptoms.

Indeed, Asperger syndrome in adults does not mean they cannot live a normal life, nor they can build good relationships. Adults with this disorder can still lead a good life, get a career, live independently and can get married. However, the challenge in dealing with their behavior may remain. With proper cognitive therapy, support and good education, they will eventually learn to cope up with the symptoms.

In fact, most sufferers of this disorder have average to above average intelligence and they may develop an intense interest on a particular thing or passion like music and math and may excel on it.

If you have a partner with Asperger syndrome, you may also need to have practical and emotional support especially when you already have kids. You have to understand that they find it difficult to understand your feelings and may not be able to support you in what you need so you have to plan everything out and how you can deal with it especially when it comes to parenting.

Finding careers for adults with Asperger

syndrome may also require careful selection. Usually, they can get a career which requires visual thinking like careers in design or drafting. They may also get a successful career in music or those that may require good mathematics such as accounting.

To help you deal with Asperger syndrome in adults, it is also helpful to find social training sessions to help the sufferer cope up with his difficulty in social interaction. As a partner, you may also need counseling and guidance in order to deal with this disorder and help you understand your partner well.

## LIVING WITH YOUR ADULT CHILD

There are many issues involved in dealing with Asperger's syndrome in adults that you would not necessarily have with other adult children. The issue of readiness to live alone at 18 or 21 is one of them.

Many young adults without neurological disabilities are also living with their parents after graduating from college or high school as well. The press has even given them the name "boomerang kids." Still, living with your adult Asperger's child does have its special challenges. So how do you make sure it works for both of you?

## 1. Set clear boundaries

To start with, you need to set clear boundaries and rules as to the living situation, and what will be expected of all people in the household. This is a good idea no matter which you are living with. But if you are dealing with an adult child with Asperger's syndrome this has extra importance. Why? Because these adults crave clarity and direction. They completely flounder without it. They do not have the ability to read between the lines and understand what is expected of them. You have to spell it out.

## 2. Make rules clear

You can save yourself a lot of resentment in the future by making these rules clear ahead of time. Do you want your adult child to help with the chores around the house? Pay rent? Come home by a certain time of night? Limit the number of people they have over? Then tell them in very explicit terms.

Never assume "Oh, a reasonable person would know to put the dishes away without being told" or "Anyone would know it's impolite to have friends over after 11 pm" or whatever it may be -- and then get mad at your child when they break these invisible rules! Common sense is not the strength of a person with Asperger's syndrome. Mostly, they march according to their logic, which makes perfect sense to them. But if you explain to them why you want something a done a certain way or why a certain thing is important to you, then they are perfectly capable of, and usually even eager to, follow the rules.

3. Pay attention to emotional maturity, anxiety, and level of detail

It can be a hard transition for anyone who is leaving the relatively sheltered world of education to whatever comes next. When dealing with Asperger's syndrome in adults, though, going from a structured existence where there were clear goals and ways to accomplish them to an aimless existence in which none of this exists can be very hard. You also have to remember that emotional maturity levels of this age group will be behind typical kids, due to the nature of developmental disabilities.

## THE EXPERIENCE OF A YOUNG WOMAN

One young woman reveals the following about her experiences living with her parents after college.

When I lived at my parents' house after college, I was an extremely frustrated person. I had absolutely nothing to do with my time, and no way to get out of the house except for perhaps once a week. I didn't drive, and we lived far from town. I had no control over my life whatsoever.

I would go to my parents for sympathy but they'd just get mad at me. They would go out for dinner, and I'd spend the whole evening resenting that they were able to leave the house and I wasn't. When they'd come home late at night, they'd ask me why I hadn't done the dishes or some other chore, and I'd explode at them about how lucky they were and get mad at them for asking me to help.

It is clear that I had very little emotional maturity at that time. I was drowning in self-pity and didn't even realize it, and it made me a pretty selfish person at that time in my life. I had no way to feel like I had any control over my life, so had no way to get out of it.

I should have been grateful for a place to stay and helped out around the house in return, but no one had made it clear to me that this was what I was expected to do. And I was so deep in my own feelings of remorse for the life I wanted to have that I couldn't see it.

WHAT WOULD HELP THIS SITUATION?

In retrospect, there are a few things that would have made this situation better. When she came home from college, there should have been an in-depth, very detailed explanation of "We're glad to help you out for a little bit and let you stay here, but we expect some things in return. We know the (circumstances of your life that brought you to this place) are very hard, but we still need you to help out." Then list the specific chores she would be responsible for, or at least the specific things she should make a point to look for to see if they needed to be done. Make a chart. Make it visual, make it stick, and most of all, do it at a time when no one is defensive and it's being done out of love rather than resentment.

## The method of communication matters for adults with Asperger's Syndrome

Telling someone to do something in a tone of voice that implies you are angry at them will not have the effect you want when dealing with Asperger's syndrome in adults. Adults with Asperger's syndrome are very sensitive to emotion, despite not always being able to display it.

They will pick up on the anger in your tone

and be so overwhelmed by it that they will not be able to process what you are saying. The anger is scary to them and makes them go into "survival mode" or at least get very defensive. This takes all their mental energy, and they will totally not remember what you are saying.

Therefore, the mistake will be repeated again and again and again until tensions escalate to unbearable levels. Each party is just trying to do what seems right to them, but both parties fail to see that a lack of proper communication is causing all this resentment. It matters how you communicate.

Be aware of each other's emotions, and pay attention to detail

The level of detail also matters. Telling your adult child to "help around the house more" is a very ambiguous statement. Adults with Asperger's syndrome do not do well with ambiguous statements. Telling them "You should know to do this without us asking" is not helpful either. The feelings of guilt and inadeMuacy that it creates gets in the way of any helpful message getting across. If they knew to do it, they would be doing it. Most adults with Asperger's syndrome are eager to please.

Be specific on what chores you want to be done when, how many friends is a "few," what time "by night" means, or any other ambiguous statement. You may think "They're so smart, they should know this stuff," but remember, adults with Asperger's syndrome have uneven abilities. They seem very smart in some areas, but can be Muite clueless in others.

In most cases, it is not a case of laziness. It's a case of having no idea what one is supposed to do or having too much emotional baggage or anxiety to pay attention to anything but the thoughts in their head. In either case, specific direction can work wonders.

## A PARENT'S GUIDE TO ASPERGERS SYNDROME

Kids with Aspergers don't usually share the withdrawn isolation of children with autism and will openly, but often very awkwardly, approach and engage others in social situation. However, their inability to see things through others eyes, and the tendency to go overboard going on and on about their latest obsession, makes them appear selfish, uncaring and insensitive toward other people. This is not necessarily true, they just don't realize how they are perceived or that other people have different interests and feelings than they do.

Many of the children with Aspergers will actually memorize reactions in specific social situations, and recite definitions or examples of emotion, but have a very hard time acting on any of that knowledge in a real situation. Or they will use a rigid application of the specific social rules they have memorized. This can come across as forced eye contact, or the plastered on smile, or laughing at the wrong time. They want friends and do seek out social contact, but over the years their failures in these situations can be devastating.

Kids with Aspergers will sometimes develop very focused and intense interest in something or some activity, that will completely dominate their time and their life, almost to the exclusion of everything else, and they will try to draw whoever they can into the same interest. This is usually seen as normal childhood interest and behavior at first until the obsessive qualities become apparent and problems relating to anything or anyone else starts happening.

Diagnosis

The diagnosis uses the identification of the stereotypical and repetitive behaviors as a central part of how it is diagnosed, but confirmation is done by ruling out anything else that can cause the same symptoms. The motor behaviors that are observed are things like the hand flapping or twisting, complex whole-body movements and walking on tiptoes, repeating the same word or sound over and over again are all typical repetitive behaviors of AS.

Other Issues

Your child may display symptoms that aren't a part of an Aspergers Syndrome diagnosis, but still, affect the child and your whole family. They may have perception difficulties, and problems with fine or gross motor skills, handling emotions, and difficulty sleeping. Many kids on the spectrum (Autism Spectrum) have trouble with SI, or Sensory Integration, and can be overly sensitive or under sensitive to sound light, touch, texture, taste, smell, pain, temperature and other things that stimulate the senses. It may feel soft and nice to you, but to them, it can be actually painful.

Children with Aspergers are more likely to have sleep problems, including difficulty in falling asleep, waking up often at night, and early morning awakenings. Aspergers is also associated with alexithymia, which means having problems identifying and describing one's emotions. My daughter certainly has emotions and feelings, but she has no idea how to describe them or even what they are, or why they are there. Very frustrating.

Special education

Children with AS may require special education services because of their social and behavioral difficulties, although many attend regular education classes. Teens and tween with Aspergers may have difficulty with self-care, organization, and disturbances in a social and romantic relationship. They are usually very smart, but the inability to properly express and the awkwardness of social contact keep many from leaving home as adults, although some gain independence in work and domicile, even marrying and raising a family. Teen and preteen years are hard enough on kids without social difficulties but can be very traumatic for a kid dealing with Aspergers.

Coexisting conditions

Anxiety with AS is very common and is usually centered on change or transition. That is why a consistent schedule is so important. Anxiety and stress during social situations is inevitable because of the constantly changing nature of humans and relationships and situations, there isn't a single right thing to do in every situation. Stress and anxiety will show up usually as a behavior, such as withdrawal, an obsession, hyperactivity, or even aggressive or oppositional behavior.

Depression, and other mood disorders can be the end result of the constant stress and frustration of failing to properly socialize and make friends. Medication and behavior therapy can be used to deal with co-existing problems such as anxiety, depression, inattention, obsessive compulsion, and aggression.

Getting the family involved by helping them to understand what is going on with their child or brother or sister, will have a big impact on the child's future. It will also help with being able to deal with everything that is involved in dealing with a child with Aspergers Syndrome and bring some semblance of normalcy back to the family. Getting help early and involving the whole family as a built-in support system has the best effect on long term outcomes for a child with Aspergers Syndrome.

# CHAPTER FIVE
# ASPERGER SYNDROME IN CHILDREN

Some ways you can develop an understanding of Asperger symptoms in children is to know how to identify the traits and behavioral patterns that Aspergers children possess. Many children with Asperger symptoms are usually above average in their level of intelligence. The majority of children with Asperger's syndrome have above average intellectual skills, but the children usually have trouble with the interpretation of human relationships.

Some children with Asperger's syndrome may find themselves being intensely preoccupied with one task. Sometimes conversations between a child with Asperger's syndrome is a one-sided conversation due to the child not taking interest in any forms of feedback. Older children with Asperger's syndrome can enjoy focused interest clubs such as stamp or coin collection types of clubs.

At times, the child with Asperger symptoms may appear uncaring, but this is not done deliberately, as many children may exhibit such mannerisms because it is difficult for them to understand the social behaviors that society expects of them. It is possible to encourage and even teach social skills to children with Asperger symptoms. If you try to teach social skills, you should be patient as it can be quite a long process. Parents are encouraged to take an interest during the social training aspect of Asperger's children.

Teaching social skills can be done through visual aids that can help Aspergers children to learn how to listen to others as well as remain silent when others are talking. This would encourage a two-way conversation rather than a one-way conversation.

Dealing with Asperger symptoms in children can be difficult; however, unlike other children, they re⬚uire routine as well as structure in their life.

## CHILDREN WITH ASPERGERS SYNDROME

Many children with Asperger's syndrome can attend regular school, as the majority of children with this syndrome possess advanced intellectual and language development. The only difference is that the children with this syndrome are more likely to experience social problems relative to the integration re⬚uired with other pupils at regular schools.

In social situations, some people may perceive a child with Asperger's syndrome to being aloof or indifferent, but technically this is a result of the syndrome and is not a purposeful action.

If left unchecked, children with this syndrome may be unable to fully develop the appropriate social and peer relationships they need to prosper later on in adulthood. With Aspergers, many children with the syndrome are not usually able to qualify for supportive services due to their relative good behavior.

Other forms of support and training are essential in order to integrate children into society as social beings. Since children with Asperger's syndrome tend to struggle with the social aspects of life, social interaction training and support is important in order to advance such children into society.

Some Symptoms of Children with Aspergers Syndrome include:

Difficulties in Social Situations

The child has a strong dislike in social interactions

They avoid eye contact at all costs

Are preoccupied with one specific subject or hobby

Socially withdrawn

Serious lack of interest in making friendships

## DIFFICULTIES COMMUNICATING

Child is unable to provide the right social clues

Body language very difficult to decipher

Unable to let other people take turns in talking

Extensive trouble in starting conversations or maintaining themselves

Child may possess an advanced form of speech for their age

Flat speech that may lack pitch and tone

At a younger age, the child may excessively repeat words or phrases while speaking

DIFFICULTIES WITH MOTOR SKILLS

Difficulties with posture and facial expressions

Clumsiness and uncoordinated movements

Repetitive movements of other body parts such as flapping hands and fingers

Delayed motor development

IDENTIFYING SYMPTOMS OF ASPERGERS SYNDROME IN CHILDREN

Aspergers Syndrome is inside the spectrum of Autism disorders and it is generally accepted as a form of high functioning Autism. If your child has Aspergers then a few symptoms that they present may be very different from Asperger's symptoms that you have witnessed in others. It really is even more difficult to ascertain the level of Aspergers in your child if they are yet to achieve school age as their only real social interaction could have been with close relatives and buddies.

HOW CAN YOU TELL IF YOUR CHILD HAS ASPERGERS?

Aspergers Syndrome was discovered in just before 1945 and was named pediatrician and psychiatrist that discovered it, Hans Asperger. Unfortunately, the clarification of the disorder was not widely accepted until 1981, so telling if your kid has Aspergers can be ?uite a difficult task but there are a few general tips that you could evaluate to better your understanding whether or not your child is showing some symptoms of Aspergers:

Aspergers Symptoms can range from very mild to extremely severe. Youngsters with Aspergers generally have difficulty with even tiniest amount of change to any routines and prefer consistency in everything. Any change to a routine might cause the child being reduced into tantrums.

A lot of the time Youngsters with Aspergers will be referred to as 'Little Professors' as Asperger's sufferers will have normal intelligence but often they'll display a high level of skill in a particular area.

All Asperger's sufferers have a big problem with social interactions. Kids that suffer from Aspergers will desperately desire to play with their friends however they struggle with the capability to interact and can often be seen left at the side of games within the playground. You should note that whilst from your point of view that may be seen as extremely sad, they could well not recognize the social stigma 'left out' as much as somebody that does not suffer from Aspergers.

Children with AS (Asperser's Syndrome) have a tendency to see the world in a different way to non AS sufferers. It's not that they are being rude or odd on purpose.

Aspergers Children will come across as quite uncompassionate and never sympathetic but this again is not on purpose, they only don't realize that it is crucial or expected in society.

Many will not even with others however, this is not the case Asperger's sufferers. Some kids with Aspergers will talk in unusual tones or have exceptionally fast speech patterns however, not all experience this.

If your little one is very sound, light or different types of food this can also be a signal of Aspergers.

## HOW DO I KNOW IF MY CHILD HAS IT?

Are you the parent of a young child that may have some signs of autism but does not have a lot of them? Have you been told by a Doctor or special education personnel that your child may have Aspergers Syndrome (AD)? Would you like to learn about the characteristics of the disorder so that you can pursue private evaluations? In this part, we will be discussing the characteristics of this syndrome so that you will be able to advocate for appropriate educational services for your child.

This disorder was initially described by Hans Asperger in 1944. He found a number of cases whose clinical characteristics were similar to autism but differed in the fact that the speech was less commonly delayed, motor clumsiness was much more common, and initial cases seem to only occur in boys.

In 1994 The American Psychiatric Association added Asperger's syndrome to it's Diagnostic and Statistical Manual of Mental Disorders, often referred to as the DSM IV.

It is listed by itself in its own category and not under the autism umbrella but under the broader Pervasive Developmental Disorder.

CHARACTERISTICS OF THIS DISORDER ARE:

1. Major impairment in social interaction which may show in lack of empathy, difficulty with spontaneity, difficulty in developing friendships with peers, ability to show social reciprocity which is back and forth communication, and impairments in eye contact, posture, and gestures.

2. Restricted repetitive patterns of behavior, interests, and activities. This can be shown by preoccupation with one area of interest that is abnormal in intensity or

focus.

The child may be very inflexible when it comes to daily routines or rituals, and also may show an extreme preoccupation with a part of objects.

3. While a child with AD acquires language skills without delay, they often have abnormalities in how they use language.

4. Children with this disorder may also have unusual sensory experiences, like sensitivities to light or sound. This disorder is called Sensory Integration Dysfunction.

5. Motor clumsiness is another characteristic of this disorder. Children with this disorder may be delayed in learning skills that require motor dexterity such as riding a bike or opening a jar.

6. Children with this disorder do not show a significant delay in cognitive development.

7. Some children with this disorder are

extremely bright with very high IQ's.

The best way to determine if a child has Aspergers is to have your child evaluated by a competent trained professional such as a Neuropsychologist or a Clinical Psychologist. Many school psychologists are not trained to diagnose this disorder, so it may be best to have your child privately tested.

Two of the instruments that may be used are the Autism Diagnostic Interview-Revised (ADI R), and the Autism Diagnostic Observation Schedule (ADOS).

It is important to note however that this disorder may be Co-Morbid with other disorders. This means that the child may have other disorders as well. These may be ADHD, Bi-Polar Disorder, Learning Disabilities, or Obsessive Compulsive Disorder. The earlier treatment for this disorder and comorbid disorders, the better it will be for your child. Appropriate special education services can help your child be ready for post-school learning and independent living, as the Individuals with Disabilities Education Act (IDEA) requires!


## TESTED WAYS TO HELP CHILDREN WITH ASPERGER SYNDROME

Asperger Syndrome is one of several autism spectrum disorders. It is characterized by problems in social interaction, although bad motor skills are also a common condition of Asperger Syndrome. Treatment for Asperger Syndrome varies with each child. There is no medication to treat a child with Asperger's, but there are treatments to help with the symptoms of the condition.

The treatments can vary because different things will work for different children. Just because one treatment works for one child that has Asperger Syndrome doesn't mean it will work for another. Here is a look at the different treatments a child with Asperger

Syndrome can have:

Social Skills Training: Children suffering from Asperger's have a hard time distinguishing facial expressions and voice tone. They don't understand the different meanings and will take everything said literally. These children will be taught the differences between facial expressions and voice tone and will help them understand jokes and sarcasm. Children with Asperger Syndrome usually have a difficult time making eye contact. Giving them training in social skills will help them interact with other people and other children better, making the social setting a lot easier for them.

Cognitive Behavior Therapy: This type of therapy helps children recognize a bad situation before it happens. Many children with Asperger's usually have high anxiety and this type of therapy will teach them how to reduce stress. Normally, the child will have a meltdown or throw a temper tantrum when something doesn't go their way. This type of therapy helps children to cope and handle situations better, reducing the number of outbursts.

Parental Education: Children aren't the only ones who can go through training. Parents can also take training classes to learn how to deal with their children who have Asperger Syndrome. Some of the tips that parents are taught are to use a reward system with your child. The reward system shows the child that by remaining calm will have its benefits. However, this training also shows parents how to handle children when they have outbursts.

Medication: There isn't a specific medicine that will treat Asperger's, but there are prescriptions to treat symptoms. Children can take anxiety or depression medication. Unfortunately, these pills may have side effects and you have to monitor your children closely. Check to see how they are responding and if their behavior is more unusual. Some children may also have a difficult time sleeping. Children with Asperger Syndrome can be given sleeping sills or some type of sedative to help them at night.

Positive Reinforcement: Children with Asperger Syndrome can do well with the parents and other authority figures giving positive reinforcement. By showing them what they need to do and support them through their endeavors, children with Asperger Syndrome can maintain independent lifestyles.

Children with Asperger Syndrome don't have to be left behind. They have can have normal lives and with proper treatments, children with Asperger Syndrome don't have to suffer. There are no magic pills or treatments that are going to cure Asperger's, but there are ways to help reduce the symptoms. Talk to your doctor about the different treatment options to help your child in social settings.

## SEEKING SUPPORT

When it comes to taking care of children with Asperger's syndrome, it is probable that you will need to be both uncomplaining and resourceful, as every child is unique and it might be necessary to experiment with a plethora of tactics before recognizing the one that works the best. While it is a good idea to discuss with qualified general practitioners, psychologists, and school administrators, don't forget that you know your child best, therefore you also need to use your own intelligence and skills of observation. Up next are some healing methods for Aspergers that might work optimally for your child.

Because of their learning style, many children with Aspergers have difficulty learning in a normal classroom setting, even though they are extremely bright. You may need to talk to your child's teachers and the school administrators to get your child extra help. A concise, step by step learning method works best for children with Asperger's as well as having both verbal and visual instructions. They may be labeled as a slow learner but this is seldom true; all they need is a teacher who knows how their mind works. So part of treating a child with Aspergers is making sure that they get any academic help they need. Since public schools are required by law to provide resources to children with special needs, don't be afraid to talk to your school and make sure they are doing everything they can to help your child learn. Even though common expectations are that there is a drug to treat everything, there is no specific medication for Asperger's syndrome. But there are medications available that can help treat particular symptoms related to this condition.

Many children with Aspergers also suffer from other conditions that can include ADD, bipolar disorder, and depression. Medication, in some cases, has been used to effectively control these symptoms. No one set of medications will work in all cases because of the varied symptoms of Aspergers. So, as far as treating kids with Aspergers, there is no single drug for it, but medication may be prescribed to help with certain symptoms.

You can often get a great deal of help from other parents of children with Asperger's syndrome. There may be support groups in your area. Be sure and check out forums and online groups. Information and tips can be found here, as well as moral support.

If you have just discovered your child's condition, you may be able to find a parent with an older child with Asperger's syndrome who can give you advice. With all the options available, your child's doctor or psychologist may not be aware of all the treatment options, and you may learn other options through here.

Reach out through all the information available and find others who are familiar with this situation. Other parents can be a huge help when dealing with Asperger's syndrome.

You can do a variety of things to alleviate a child who has Aspergers and the particular strategy you use needs to be based on the child's distinctive needs. In a lot of situation, you can discover helpful healing methods to aid with the more challenging syndromes. While your child will always be a bit unusual, there are no grounds for him or her not being able to lead a cheery or industrious life. The cures for Aspergers that we have been researching can assist you in determining the optimal selections.

## ROUTINES FOR CHILDREN WITH ASPERGERS SYNDROME

Parents of children with Aspergers want to find the best treatment options for this condition. Aspergers cannot be cured however, because it is not a disease. When doctors treat Aspergers, they are actually helping the child to function better in areas where they are experiencing problems. The following are some Asperger's treatments that can be helpful in many cases.

Children with Aspergers are affected greatly by any change in their routine, therefore it is key to keep as much stability in their life as possible. Assigning times for even simple tasks like free time, homework and mealtime will help give them structure in their routine. Raising children can be done either this way or with a more freer style. Regardless of your preference, too much flexibility for a child with Aspergers will just confuse them. Life will be less stressful for them with a constant routine.

Be sure to discuss your child's Asperger's syndrome with their school psychologist. Children with Aspergers can function at high levels in school, as long as you work with the school and determine what services they have available. If your child has any areas of difficulty, either with certain academic subjects or fitting in socially, the school authorities can sometimes help. From the principals to the teachers, take the time to get to know each as much as possible. For parents of children with Aspergers, this is more important than the average parent.

This way the school is more likely to keep you informed regarding the progress your child is making, and you can tell them about any areas of concern. The adjusting period can be difficult for children with Aspergers, but once past this hurdle, many do fine in the average classroom. There are a few that can never get past the adjustment phase though. Adjusting may be difficult due to your child's particular symptoms or even the school in your area. Some kids will bully children with Aspergers making it hard for them to fit in and adjust to their surroundings. Homeschooling can be an option if this is the case, or perhaps a program to teach you and your child special skills, or even a special school. The point is, if the school your child is going to isn't helping him or her to adjust well to life, you should seek an alternative or at least additional help.

There are many ways to help children with Aspergers learn the necessary skills to function in society. Today you can find lots of options in the form of programs, treatments, organizations, both in your area and online. You and your child can find the right plan with just a little research.

# REAL STRATEGIES TO DEAL WITH ASPERGERS BEHAVIOR

Disciplining children displaying Asperger characteristic behavior will often require an approach which is somewhat unique to that of other children. Finding the balance between understanding the needs of a child with Aspergers and discipline which is age appropriate and situationally necessary is achievable when applying some simple but effective strategies. These strategies can be implemented both at home or in more public settings.

## General Behavior Problems

Traditional discipline may fail to produce the desired results for children with Asperger's syndrome, primarily because they are unable to appreciate the consequences of their actions.

Consequently, punitive measures are apt to

exacerbate the type of behavior the punishment is intended to reduce, whilst at the same time giving rise to distress in both the child and parent.

At all times the emotional and physical wellbeing of your child should take priority. Often this will necessitate removing your child from a potentially distressing situation as soon as possible. Consider maintaining a diary of your child's behavior with a view to ascertaining patterns or triggers. Recurring behavior may be indicative of a child taking some satisfaction in receiving the desired response from peers, parents or teachers.

For example, a child with Aspergers may come to understand that hurting another child in the class will result in his being removed from class, notwithstanding the associated conseℚuence to his peer. The solution may not be most effectively rooted in punishing the child for the behavior, or even attempting to explain the situation from the perspective of their injured peer, but by treating the root cause behind the motivation for the misbehavior...for example, can the child be made more comfortable in class so that they will not want to leave it?

One of the means to achieve this may be to focus on the positive. Praise for good behavior, and reinforcement can assist. The use of encouraging verbal cues delivered in a calm tone are likely to elicit more beneficial responses than the harsher verbal warnings which might be effective on children who are not displaying some sort of Asperger characteristic. If necessary, when giving directions to cease a type of misbehavior, these should also be couched as positives rather than negatives. For example, rather than telling a child to stop hitting his brother with the ruler, the child should be directed to put the ruler down.

Obsessive or fixated behavior

Almost all children go through periods of development where they become engrossed in one subject matter or another, but children with Aspergers often display obsessive and repetitive characteristics, which can have significant implications for behavior.

For example, if an Asperger's child becomes fixated upon reading a particular story each night, they may become distressed if this regime is not adhered to, or if the story is interrupted. Again, the use of a behavior diary can assist in identifying fixations for your child. Once fixation is identified, it is important to set appropriate boundaries for your child. Providing a structure within which your child can explore the obsession can assist in then keeping the obsession within reasonable limits, without the associated angst which might otherwise arise through such limitations. For example, tell your child that they may watch their favorite cartoon for half an hour after dinner, and make a clear time for that in their routine.

It is appropriate to utilize the obsession to motivate and reward your child for good behavior. Always ensure any reward associated with positive behavior is ground immediately to assist the child in recognizing the nexus between the two.

A particularly useful technique to try to develop social reciprocity is to have your child talk for five minutes about a particularly favored topic after they have listened to you talk about an unrelated topic. This serves to help your child understand that not everyone shares their enthusiasm for their subject matter.

BRIDGING THE GAP BETWEEN ASPERGERS AND DISCIPLINE AND OTHER SIBLINGS

For siblings without Asperger's syndrome, the differential and what at times no doubt appears to be preferential treatment received by an Aspergers sibling can give rise to feelings of confusion and frustration. Often they will fail to understand why their brother or sister apparently seems free to behave as they please without the normal constraints placed upon them.

It is important to explain to siblings, or peers of Asperger's children and encourage open discussion about the disorder itself. Encouragement should extend to the things siblings can do to assist the Aspergers child, and this should be positively reinforced through acknowledgment when it occurs.

Sleep difficulties

Aspergers Children are renounced for experiencing sleep problems. Children with Aspergers may have lesser sleep re uirements, and as such are more likely to become anxious about sleeping, or may find they become anxious when waking during the night or early in the morning.

Combat your child's anxiety by making their bedrooms a place of safety and comfort. Remove or store items which might be prone to injure your child if they decide to wander at night. Include in the behavioral diary a record of your child's sleep patterns. It may assist your child if you keep a list of their routine, including dinner, bath time, story and bed, in order to provide structure. Include an image or symbol of them waking in the morning to provide assurance as to what will happen. Social stories have proven to be a particularly successful tactic in decreasing a child's anxiety by providing clear instructions on how part of their day is likely to play out.

At School

Another Asperger characteristic is that children will often experience difficulty during parts of the school day which lack structure. If left to their own devices their difficulties with social interaction and self-management can result in anxiety. The use of a buddy system can assist in providing direction, as can the creation of a timetable for recess and lunch times. These should be raised with class teachers and implemented with their assistance.

Explain the concept of free time to your child, or consider providing a separate purpose or goal for your child during such time, such as reading a book, or helping to set up paint and brushes for the afternoon tasks.

In public

Children with Aspergers can become overwhelmed to the point of distress by even a short sojourn in public. The result is that many parents with Aspergers simply seek to avoid as much as possible situations where their child is exposed to the public. Whilst expedient, it may not offer the best long term solution to your child, and there are strategies to assist with outings.

Consider providing your child with an iPod, or have the radio on in the car to block out other sounds and stimuli. Prepare a social story or list explaining to the child a trip to the shops, or doctor. Be sure to include on the list your return home. Consider giving your child a task to complete during the trip, or having them assist you. At all times, maintaining consistency when dealing with Aspergers and discipline is key. It pays to ensure that others involved in your child's care are familiar with your strategies and techniques, such as those outlined above, and are able to apply them.

Most importantly, don't hesitate to seek support networks for parents with Asperger's syndrome, and take advantage of the wealth of knowledge those who have dealt with the disorder before you have developed. The assistance you can gain from these and other resources can assist you in developing important strategies to deal with problems with Aspergers in a manner most beneficial to your child.

## THE IMPORTANCE OF SOCIALIZING FOR CHILDREN WITH ASPERGERS

If you have a child that has been diagnosed with Asperger's syndrome, you want to find the best treatments available. Aspergers cannot be cured however, because it is not a disease. When doctors treat Aspergers, they are actually helping the child to function better in areas where they are experiencing problems. Others have found the following treatments for Aspergers to be effective.

Children with Aspergers often have problems communicating and socializing with their peers, so social skills is an important area of treatment. Very often, kids with Aspergers have to learn basic skills of interacting that most people take for granted. For example, their speech pattern often sounds unnatural, so they can learn to talk in a more natural sounding way. Normal body language and making eye contact need to be taught to them as well. And because they often have trouble with sarcasm and tone of voice, they need to learn how to understand some forms of humor. Because each child will have different needs, the type of treatment needs to be aimed at the individual child. It is valuable to teach these skills to a child with Aspergers because it allows them to relate to others better.

You have to be alert for any negative reaction triggers when treating children with Aspergers. Each child will have a different trigger and it could be anything. Other people will hardly notice these things, but since children with Aspergers are wired differently, they may react to certain lights, sounds, tastes or even feelings. If you find that a certain room agitates your child, check out the lighting in the room or be aware of any noises that may be different. You have to learn to recognize these things since they can be very disturbing for children with Aspergers.

Parents of children of Asperger's syndrome often find help from other parents. Look for support groups in your area. Online groups and forums are another great resources to look at. These offer moral support as well as information and tips.

Often parents who have older children with Aspergers have years of experience they can share with the parent who just discovered their child's condition. Other treatment options may be discovered through these resources, that even your doctor or child's psychologist have not thought of. With all the information available to us these days, it is nice to find someone who is in a similar circumstance. Other parents can be a huge help when dealing with Asperger's syndrome. Because

Aspergers is still being studied, even the experts have a lot to learn about this condition. Be vigilant to see which treatments are helping your child with Aspergers and which ones aren't Keeping the above suggestions in mind and working closely with a qualified doctor will help you help your child adjust better to the world around him.

## HOW TO HELP YOUR ASPERGERS CHILD MAKE FRIENDS?

It is no secret that children can be cruel and a child that does not appear to fit in can be the subject of taunting and ridicule. This present a major problem for the child and his parents as the child will have trouble making and retaining friends and other social interactions, and the child with Aspergers Syndrome can be adversely affected.

First of all, please understand that just because your child has Aspergers does not mean that they are intellectually limited. Various studies, in fact, have indicated that children with Aspergers are actually very smart, many times being intellectually superior to their peers of the same age group. Unfortunately, the social interaction part of their maturity has fallen behind the rest of their maturing process, which presents the parents with another challenge along the same lines. In other words, they are probably not intellectually challenged, but simply "socially challenged", and the best thing you can do as parents is to work with them to help them overcome that aspect.

One of the best things you can do as parents is to do role-playing activities or scenarios which would reflect a natural social environment such as another child's birthday party or pool party or similar setting. Work with the child to help them understand how to join in with the playground games, how to converse with their playmates, and what is and is not expected of them in this type of setting. Helping them to become comfortable in this type of setting can go a long ways towards helping them fit in when they participate in actual events with their peers.

Children with Aspergers will face internal anxiety if they cannot accept their current surroundings. Try to teach them not to obsess about objects or any preferred items or activities. Work with them to find out what calms them so that anxiety can be subdued and controlled. Normal everyday life at school can present its own unique set of challenges since social interaction is a normal part of school life. Be sure to let the teachers know about the Aspergers in your child so that they can make accommodations for them as they are able to. Most schools are happy to work with you and your child in this respect, but it will take effort on both parts. Work with your child at home to help them become comfortable with social interactions, perhaps starting with just one friend on a one-to-one basis and then increasing to more friends. Put them in an environment, even in your role-playing, where they will see and recognize success, instead of putting them in a situation where failure is inevitable.

Children with Aspergers need to be given extra chances to make and retain friends, build social networks, and understand what is acceptable for interacting with others. If you can work with them in a role-playing environment, it will be easier for them to learn these skills. Do not force them, but rather be positive and supportive so that they will not dread any future social interactions.

HOW BASEBALL CAN BENEFIT A CHILD WITH

# ASPERGER'S SYNDROME

## STORY FROM A PARENT

As a parent of a nine-year-old with Asperger's Syndrome, I can share in the wonder, joy, amazement, and often the frustration of seeing my child develop and the challenges he faces each day.

Asperger's is considering highly functioning autism. A child with this particular disorder is considered high functioning because their cognitive and linguistic faculties are often very much on par with their peers.

However, children with Asperger's Syndrome can have severe challenges in the area of social interaction. In addition, they can exhibit extreme instances of repetitive behaviors and obsessive focus on certain routines. Lack of empathy, poor communication skills, difficulty with social adjustment, trouble with basic life skills, and physical clumsiness are other aspects of the disorder.

Recently, my son expressed great interest in baseball. After playing a baseball video game at home, he began to obsess over baseball eＱuipment, baseball uniforms, watching baseball on television, how runners advance to a base after hitting the ball, where players would throw the ball during a play, etc. Rather than deter his obsession, I decided to embrace it and nurture it in a healthy way.

Over time, I suggested that he might want his own baseball glove and baseball, so I purchased both for him. Before long, we began to practice throwing and catching. From there, his focus moved to hit, so I purchased a bat, and we began to practice batting.

I also purchased a baseball hat, pants, and shirt, so he could have his own uniform. We began to discuss how kids could play baseball on a team, just like the players he saw on television. At first, I could tell he was hesitant about the idea, but gradually, he warmed up to it.

Ultimately, my son told me he wanted to try to play baseball on a team. He did this without any solicitation on my part. It was a very natural request related to his introduction to the things he already liked to do. By being able to obsess about the details, he gradually warmed up to the bigger picture.

Of course, we signed him up for a team. He has a great coach that is fully aware of his condition and works well with him. Being on the team provides great structure. My son understands that there are rules that must be followed. Though social interaction is still a challenge, he does reach out to this teammates on a more regular basis, and he operates more independently.

He understands that in order to play baseball, a baseball player must dress before a practice or a game, for example. For a child with Asperger's Syndrome, baseball can be great therapy. Nurturing an obsession and allowing it to develop into a more normal interest is key.

SHOULD I TELL MY CHILD THAT S/HE HAS ASPERGER'S?

For the answer to this question, I turned to some information from a renowned expert psychologist in the area of Asperger's syndrome. "The answer is a resounding 'Yes.'" according to Dr. Attwood. After many years of clinical experience, he has found that explaining the diagnosis to the child with Asperger's syndrome is extremely important.

By giving the child an accurate picture of Asperger's syndrome, you will be helping prevent inappropriate coping mechanisms (which may include reactive depression, too much use of imagination to escape reality, aggression/acting out, denial).

Dr. Attwood describes an exercise he goes through with the Asperger's child and his/her parents. It's called Attribution Exercise. Picture a large whiteboard, or piece of paper. The therapist takes out this whiteboard or piece of paper and divides it into two columns. One column is called "Qualities." The other column is called "Difficulties."

There can be a different large piece of paper for different members of the family. First, the mother or father can fill out their own piece of paper, identifying his/her own ⬚ualities and difficulties.

Qualities may include the following:

Practical abilities

Knowledge

Personality

How this particular person expresses and manages their feelings

Difficulties can include any areas of growth/deficiencies (for example, this writer struggles with 'handyman' skills, and with organizational skills: just ask his wife).

After the mother/father has done his/her turn, the child with Aspergers can then do the exercise, with some support and encouragement from the parent. The therapist can comment on the child's qualities and difficulties, finding areas of commonality with the diagnostic criteria for Aspergers Syndrome. Then, s/he can explain that scientists study different patterns in behavior, and when they find those patterns, they give the pattern a name. The therapist can then explain that, over 60 years ago, a doctor in Vienna, Dr. Hans Asperger, studied children with similar characteristics, and published the first clinical description that has come to be known as Asperger's syndrome.

Next, the therapist, and you, can congratulate your child on having Asperger's syndrome. Explain that they have strengths and talents (e.g., extensive knowledge about certain subjects, ability to draw with photographic realism, attention to detail, talents in mathematics or writing), but that they also have a different way of thinking.

## EFFECTS ON RELATIONSHIP BUILDING FOR CHILDREN WITH ASPERGERS

Since the symptoms of Asperger's syndrome prevent many children with Asperger's syndrome from being emphatic towards others, they have to be trained to socially adapt and understand how their own behavior affects other people. Many times children with Asperger's syndrome have no idea about the results of their behavior towards others, this makes every relationship they may have the potential to be very difficult.

Whenever it is time to build meaningful and intimate relationships, feelings have to be expressed. The symptoms of Aspergers can make the relationship building quite difficult to build and maintain in children as well as teens and adults with Aspergers.

Getting in touch with one's feelings and being able to express such feelings at the right time can be quite difficult for young children that have Asperger's syndrome, as well as in older adults that may be married or in relationships.

Siblings to children with Asperger's syndrome can learn quite a lot with their younger brothers or sisters through joint play. Every child with Aspergers is different and is likely to have unique behaviors and characteristics. Asperger's syndrome is displayed in varying forms in each person diagnosed as having the disorder. Although this can make it difficult for schools to adjust their programs in order to suit the Childs need, it is possible with time and understanding of the condition and its implications.

Sometimes all it takes is creating special workplaces, purchasing earplugs, or breaking tasks into smaller steps so that the child with Asperger's syndrome is able to repeat the steps as reꟼuired to understand the particular assignments. Using visual aids can also help children with Aspergers learn about the importance of cultivating and understanding human development and relationship building.

There is hope to be found for children with Aspergers and with the right support and training from both health professionals, teachers and family. The symptoms of Aspergers can be greatly reduced in intensity, allowing children to thrive from childhood to adulthood while living meaningful professional and productive lives.

# CHAPTER SIX
# ASPERGER'S SYNDROME
# AND SOCIAL INTERACTION

One of the major hurdles in dealing with Asperger's Syndrome is the social difficulties that come along with it. Asperger's Syndrome affects the mind's ability to interpret the world the way everyone else does, especially when it comes to other people. Simple conversations and interactions often become a chore and thus make both the Aspie and the people they are trying to socialize with unwilling to try to overcome the difficulties. Miscommunication and misunderstandings are instead seen as insurmountable gaps in the process.

One of the more obvious social difficulties is the inability to interpret social cues. The human conversation has evolved over the millennia to include hundreds of unspoken, non-verbal contributions that are universally understood, except by people with Asperger's Syndrome.

Our facial expressions are subtle enough that a dog can read our mood and emotional state in seconds, but have no meaning at all to an Aspie. A raised eyebrow, a crooked grin, a sidelong glance, or even something as obvious as a look of shock or horror could be completely ignored or dismissed. Similarly, body language, except in the most extreme displays, will go unnoticed by someone with an autism spectrum disorder. On the other side of the conversation, the lack of those same cues could be disconcerting and strange to a regular person. There will be a lack of eye contact, seemingly inappropriate body movements, and sometimes inappropriate smiling or frowning. They will stand either too close or too far away while they talk. They will not understand politeness, and will often enter a conversation without introduction or invitation.

Another distinct pattern is a lack of empathy for those an Aspie is socializing with. They will not understand the need or use of an apology, nor will they recognize when their audience is uninterested or bored and trying to find a way out.

There are a few simple ways to help social interactions go more smoothly.

1. Always be direct - say what you mean, mean what you say.

2. Do not count on subtlety in any form. Spoken hidden meanings may be lost, and body language will not register.

3. Be understanding. As hard as it is to interact with them, understand that they're having a hard time interacting with you.

With just these few things in mind, it can make any conversation with a sufferer of Asperger's Syndrome go much better, and hopefully bridge some of those seemingly insurmountable gaps.

## ASPERGERS, COMMUNICATION, AND SOCIALIZATION

As Asperger's syndrome has increasingly been diagnosed, more treatments have as a result been developed. Categorized as a form of autism, many with Asperger's syndrome find that it is not as disabling as autism. However, kids with Aspergers do need special help in many areas, so it's good to be aware of some of the treatments that are available. Listed here are some of the better treatments for Aspergers.

Since children with Aspergers have a lot of trouble communicating and socializing, especially with their peers, one important area of treatment is social skills training. Basic interaction skills that come naturally to most children need to be taught to a child with Aspergers. Because of differences in speech patterns, for example, they often need to be taught to speak in a more normal sounding manner. In some cases, they also need to learn to make eye contact and to have what is considered normal body language. These children also have to learn how to understand things like humor, sarcasm, and tone of voice, which they often have trouble with. Treatment for social skills needs to be based on the individual child and their particular problem areas.

Teaching a child with Aspergers these kinds of skills is extremely valuable because it allows them to relate to others better. Nowadays, people often expect there to be a drug to treat every condition, but there is no specific medication for Asperger's syndrome. There are, however, medications that can be used to treat the symptoms of this condition. Children with Aspergers often also suffer from conditions like bipolar disorder and depression. In some cases, medication can help to keep these symptoms under control. People with Aspergers can have a wide range of symptoms, and any medication has to be tailored to individual cases. So, Aspergers can't be treated with a single drug but there are medications available to help with the various symptoms.

If your child has Aspergers, it is crucial for you to learn all that you can about the sickness. As there are new reports and curing options continuously being brought to light, this is a lifelong development, so it's imperative not to assume that you already are aware of everything you need to be aware of. You also need to remember not to take things personally if your child ends up acting out in a particular manner or doesn't communicate with a traditional technique. These are normal signals of Aspergers and the child isn't misbehaving this way to be troubling. On occasion, parents of a child suffering from Aspergers need counseling and therapy of their own; aside from the treatments their child is receiving, to help them face the more problematical phases of this affliction.

There are a plethora of things you can do to help a child who has Aspergers and the specific strategy you utilize should be based on the child's care needs. In most cases, you can find effective treatments to help with the more difficult symptoms. While your child will always be distinctive, there isn't any rationale that says they can't also lead a joyful and prolific life. The healing methods for Aspergers that we've been investigating can assist you in discovering the greatest choices.

# ASPERGER'S SYNDROME AND EDUCATION

Asperger syndrome is a developmental disorder that appears in the first 3 years of life and affects the brain's normal development of social and communication skills. Those with Asperger's syndrome display varying difficulties when interacting with others. Some children and adolescents have no desire to interact, while others simply do not know how.

So what should parents/carers look for when choosing a school for their Asperger's Syndrome child, or consider in their monitoring of the school environment?

Children with Asperger's Syndrome cope best in schools with small class sizes. This option is less a reality these days when Education systems worldwide are struggling to survive with less funding and increased consumer demand. However, there are many other procedures and practices you can monitor to make certain your child with

Asperger's Syndrome is being educated in an optimal setting.

What can help your Asperger's child at school - Asperger Syndrome and Education?

1. Before the school year starts, take your child to the school for a trial run.

2. Just so they can meet their teacher and learn what their day may look like.

3. This is a good time for you to introduce yourself to the teacher and let them know that you are there to help, providing just a basic overview of your child and what works best for them, as far as you know.

4. Recognize that the teacher will have a number of children to deal with and they want to help your child, but they may need to do things differently than you have at home.

5. Let the teacher know that you are willing to support your child with homework

assignments or any other projects that may come up.

6. Be an advocate for your child but don't overwhelm the school or make demands on them that make it impossible for them to care for other children as well.

7. If your child is to be mainstreamed, they are likely going to need aid with them throughout most of their mainstreamed classes.

8. This person will be there to help them with difficult work and also monitor your child for overload, allowing them the opportunity to remove your child from the classroom prior to them displaying inappropriate behavior.

9. Inappropriate behavior in the classroom is only going to make them a target for other children and it will serve them well to avoid that possibility.

FIVE THINGS TEACHERS NEED TO KNOW

1. My child needs structure and routine in order to function. Please try to keep his world as predictable as possible.

2. If there will be any sort of change in my child's classroom or routine, please notify me as far in advance as possible so that we can all work together in preparing her for it.

3. My child's difficulty with social cues, nonverbal communication, figurative language, and eye contact are part of his neurological makeup -- he is not being deliberately rude or disrespectful.

4. My child is an individual, not a diagnosis; please be alert and receptive to the things that make her unique and special.

5. Please keep the lines of communication open between our home and the school. My child needs all the adults in his life

working together.

This is just one of the many tricks, tips, and techniques that you can use to help you Asperger's child at school.

# CHAPTER SEVEN
# ASPERGER'S SYNDROME
# ON BEHAVIOR AND
# INTERESTS

Asperger's syndrome behavior is a disorder that affects the children who have some trouble in their development of languages and communication skills. This is called "Autism Spectrum Disorders". Comparing to other syndrome disorders, the Aspergers is difficult with respect to diagnosing process. Only the males will have trouble in having this disorder. Asperger's syndrome behavior is a kind of behavior that has poor intelligence in communication skills and unable to communicate with others easily. This syndrome has miserable social interactions, compulsions, some speech patterns, and other curious mannerisms. The patients with Asperger's syndrome behavior will often be given a facial expression in practice and will have a hard section of reading the body languages of others.

Some other features of this syndrome include motor delays, ineptness, a limited amount of interests and curious preoccupations. The main reason for this syndrome is the trouble of having difficulties to interact with others and try to demonstrate the fellow feelings to others. The Aspergers syndrome behavior is a neurobiological disorder of one, whose causes are not understood completely. There is no any correct treatment for the Aspergers syndrome behavior, but this can be cured by the parents who are educated in giving their children a good training, an educational interpositions, practice in social skills, communication therapy, psycho-medical aid. The children should be treated with the right ailments with some perfect medications.

The person giving the treatment for any

particular children will become his case manager during the assumption. The important thing about this syndrome is to provide aid by many people who are well known to them. The correct problem must be identified from the children and it must be cured as early as possible. The syndrome is very difficult for diagnosing.

The children having the syndrome will re？uire early interposition and moreover, they must be treated with good care by making them involved in educational and social training. The particular stress is placed on social development including the present and past problems in the interaction of having friendships and communication.

After the treatment, the children with this syndrome may not show any development in their language. They will have good grammatical skills and moreover, they will turn good with advanced vocabulary skills as soon as in their early age. They will easily interact with other people and they very easily get good communication skills to have a friendly conversation with others. Children with Asperger's syndrome behavior will gain more and be cured by doing the above treatments and education. After the treatment the children sign with above average intelligence.

## WAYS TO OVERCOME OBSESSIONS AND COMPULSIVE ASPERGER SYNDROME BEHAVIOR

Obsessions and compulsive behavior are typical problems linked with Asperger Syndrome Behavior. This is often a hallmark sign of Asperger's syndrome. These children may become fixated on a narrow subject, such as the weather, compulsive cleanness, sports statistics or other narrow concern.

## HOW TO DEAL WITH THIS ASPERGER

SYNDROME BEHAVIOR?

Ways to overcome obsessions and compulsive behavior:

1. Communication

For example, Asperger's syndrome can be explicitly taught better ways of communicating with others which will lessen their focus on obsession.

2. Cognitive behavioral therapy

3. Medications

Medications that control obsessive behavior can be tried to see if some of the obsessiveness reduces.

In some cases, it helps to turn your child's obsession with a passion that can be integrated into his or her own extracurricular or school activities. A consuming interest in a given subject can help connect your child to schoolwork or social activities, depending on the obsession and the behavior.

## ASPERGER SYNDROME BEHAVIOR - ANGER AND DEPRESSION

Part of the problem stems from a conflict between longings for social contact and an inability to be social in ways that attract friendships and relationships.

## HOW TO COPE WITH ANGER AND DEPRESSION?

1. Communication skills and healthy self-esteem. These things can create the ability to develop relationships and friendships, lessening the chances of having issues with anger or depression.

2. Anger can also come when rituals can't get accomplished or when their need for order or symmetry can't be met.

3. Cognitive-behavioral therapy. It focuses on maintaining control in spite of the frustration of not having their needs met.

While it is better to teach communication skills and self-esteem to the younger children, communication skills and friendship skills can be taught to teens or even adults that can eliminate some of the social isolation they feel. This can avert or reverse depression and anger symptoms as well as obsessions and compulsive behavior.

## ASPERGER SYNDROME BEHAVIOR

Families must, to some extent, learn to cope with compulsive behaviors on the part of their Aspergers child. It helps to learn as much as you can about the syndrome and its nuances.

Asperger Syndrome Behavior

Learn as much about your child as you can

and learn which things trigger compulsive behavior so they can be avoided. Some compulsive behavior is completely benign and is easily tolerated by everyone involved. As parents, you need to decide which kinds of behaviors should be just tolerated and which need intervention.

Do you want to know how to...cope with your child's difficult and aggressive behaviors?

Understand what is really going on inside their child's head,

How to help your child to cope better in the community and at school, and much more about Asperger Syndrome Behavior

## ASPERGER'S SYNDROME ON SPEECH AND LANGUAGE

The goal of speech therapy is to improve all aspects of communication. This includes:

comprehension, expression, sound production, and social use of language

1. Speech therapy may include sign language and the use of picture symbols

2. At its best, a specific speech therapy program is tailored to the specific weaknesses of the individual child

3. Unfortunately, it can be difficult to create a child-specific, evolving, long-term speech therapy plan (1, 3).

The National Research Council describes four aspects of beneficial speech therapy-

1. Speech therapy should begin early in a child's life and be freꞯuent.

2. Therapy should be rooted in practical experience in a child's life.

3. Therapy should encourage spontaneous communication.

4. Any communication skills learned during

speech therapy should be generalizable to multiple situations.

Thus, any speech therapy program should include practice in many different places with many different people. In order for speech therapy to be most successful, caregivers should practice speech exercises during normal daily routines in the home, school, and community. Speech therapists can give specific examples of how best to incorporate speech therapy throughout a child's day.

What's it like?

Speech therapy sessions will vary greatly depending upon the child. If the child is younger than three years old, then the speech therapist will most likely come into the home for a one-hour session. If the child is older than three, then therapy session will occur at school or in the therapist's office. If the child is school age, expect that speech therapy will include one-on-one time with the child, classroom-based activities, and consultations between the speech therapist and teachers and parents.

The sessions should be designed to engage the child in communication. The therapist will engage the child through games and toys chosen specifically for the child.

Several different speech therapy techniques and approaches can be used in a single session or throughout many sessions.

What is the theory behind it?

Children with AS not only have trouble communicating socially but often also have problems behaving. These behavioral problems are believed to be at least partially caused by the frustration associated with the inability to communicate. Speech therapy is intended to not only improve social communication skills but also teach the ability to use those communication skills as an alternative to unacceptable behavior.

Does it work?

Many scientific studies demonstrate that speech therapy is able to improve the communication skills of children with autism

1. The most successful approaches to speech therapy include: early identification, family involvement, and individualized treatment

2. There are many different approaches to speech therapy and most of them are effective. The table below lists some of the different approaches. In most cases, a speech therapist will use a combination of approaches in a program.

Asperger's Syndrome and Communication Skills

Asperger's syndrome is a form of autism

that is characterized by at least average intelligence or above (IQ=90-110+). People with Asperger's are able to speak, able to express themselves clearly in proper sentences but at the same time have trouble communicating. How can this be possible? This brief article is an introduction to the communication difficulties that accompany Asperger's syndrome.

Pragmatic Language

Pragmatic language is a form of language that helps us interact with people around us. It is not how we pronounce or articulate words and not related to stammering or stuttering. Pragmatic language is the ability to follow a conversation, understand humor and take part in the ebb and flow of chatting and talking with friends, colleagues, and acquaintances. The following things are important attributes of pragmatic language:

Attending to the setting, event, and context

that shape/direct social language

Tailoring messages to different audiences

Understanding differences in tone of voice, style of language or formality of language

Noticing the mood, point of view or "feel" of the audience

Respecting turn-taking skill in conversation

Introducing topics in a manner that is polite, respectful and not abrupt

Being able to shift smoothly from one topic to another

Keeping the context of a conversation logical, appropriate, concise and relevant

Attending to and contributing relevant information on a conversation theme

Correcting misunderstanding, asking for clarification when needed

Explaining, informing, describing or stating

an opinion

Expressing feelings and emotions, sensations, perceptions

Ability to tell jokes and understand jokes

Ability to use idioms and understand idioms

Ability to understand sarcasm

Ability to use language to persuade

Ability to monitor facial expressions, body language, and gestures

Ability to understand the symbolic or abstract message in proverbs or metaphors

People with Asperger's have difficulty in some or all of these skills and as a result, are often at odds with people around them. When you don't understand if someone is making a joke you may take it personally and feel offended or want to lash out at them in return. If you don't understand sarcasm you will miss a lot of information about the social world around you. If you can't wait your turn in a conversation you will be perceived as a bore or monopolies of conversation.

If you don't understand facial expressions you miss a lot of emotional information being conveyed by the speaker. If you don't understand body language you may use the wrong gestures in social exchange or misinterpret gestures causing you to move away, or move to close or touch when touch is not wanted.

These are just some of the communication deficits of people with Asperger's syndrome. These deficits are real but subtle and it is important for the people who know and work with someone who has Asperger's to realize that they will have difficulty in social conversation and appear odd or unusual at times in the way they use language.

People need to realize that anyone with

Asperger's syndrome will have pragmatic language deficits to one degree or another. There are programs that assist people with Asperger's to develop better pragmatic language skills and in return for better relationships with others. There are also tests that can be administered by psychologists and speech and language therapists that assess and pinpoint strengths in pragmatic language. It is important to get help when needed and not let people with Asperger's struggle through life with social language difficulties.

# CHAPTER EIGHT
# ASPERGERS SYNDROME TREATMENTS, THERAPIES AND MEDICATION.

There is not one set remedy for Asperger's syndrome. You will not find a medication that will cure a child with Aspergers. Instead, you will find several treatments to help with the problems connected with Asperger's syndrome. Here we will examine a few of the treatments employed with Asperger's syndrome.

Social skills training

Kids with Asperger's syndrome have a hard time understanding facial gestures, and tone of voice. They tend to take everything said to them very literally. They do not know when a person is joking with them. Children can be coached to recognize changes in people's voice, and what different facial gestures mean. They, in addition, need to be instructed on how to use better eye contact. This type of training can help their child to make friends. They're taught how to act around other people. Some children with Aspergers want to be around other kids, they just are unaware of how to act with them. They can be coached how to act when out shopping, or at a restaurant.

Cognitive behavior therapy

This type of therapy instructs the youngster with Asperger's syndrome to find ways to cope. They are taught ways to slim down anxiety. They learn how to spot a predicament that can result in them trouble. Then they learn methods to cope when they're in that position. Aspergers children often have a great deal of anxiety. They have a difficult time in social settings. They can have panic attacks or complete meltdowns. Cognitive therapy teaches them ways to stop the meltdowns from occurring. This therapy will teach a youngster with

Aspergers that when they feel an unwanted behavior coming near something they are able to do to stop it.

They're taught how to remove themselves from a predicament that ensures they are uneasy.

Medicine

There is no medication that will treat Aspergers. Nonetheless, there is medicine to help with a few of the symptoms of Aspergers. Many kids with Aspergers have anxiety and depression. There are treatments that can assist relieve these problems. Relieving the anxiety can help their child feel more leisurely in social settings. Drugs like these can have side effects. You will have to monitor your child's behavior while they are on the medication. Some children with Aspergers have a hard time sleeping. There are medicines to help youngster sleep.

# Being a parent education

There is training for the mothers and fathers of Asperger's children. This training incorporates ways you can handle behaviors. Learning things that can assist to calm your child down when they are having a meltdown, or anxiety attack. Mothers and fathers are taught ways of using reward systems to control behavior problems. They are taught how to manage the behaviors in the house. This helps them to deal with behaviors away too.

With these treatments, the life of an Asperger's child can be easier. If no therapy is given kids with Aspergers can have trouble with depression, and anxiety. They have such a difficult time coping with people socially they could go to alcohol or drugs to unwind them. Getting a therapy plan that works is a principal priority for your Aspergers child.

## COGNITIVE BEHAVIORAL THERAPY (CBT) AND ASPERGER SYNDROME

Asperger Syndrome cannot be cured. However, a mixture of treatments makes it possible for those diagnosed with this form of autism to manage the symptoms that negatively affect their daily life.

Most children and adults with this condition go on to lead fulfilling lives with a personalized mixture of therapy and (sometimes) medication.

One of the most popular methods for dealing with Asperger Syndrome is Cognitive Behavioral Therapy.

About CBT

Cognitive Behavioral Therapy (CBT) is goal-oriented and proactive, where the therapist and patient work together to find a strategy for handling specific problems. This is different from regular talk-based therapy in that it goes beyond psychological assessment to hammering out particular patterns of distress, maladaptive thinking, and so forth, and working on ways to solve them. Developing coping mechanisms, positive thinking, and effective behaviors are such solutions.

How it can help?

CBT can help those with Asperger Syndrome manage their obsessive interests and reliance on routines; it's also useful in developing methods for improving social interaction. It does this by having the patient identify the anxiety that comes with relying on routines-or, in the case of socialization, what parts of conversation and relationships confuse them. After these problems are identified, the therapist and patient work together to create exercises and step-by-step instructions for reducing anxiety and knowing what to do in social situations.

Because it demands the patient to get in touch with his or her feelings and work through negative emotions, CBT has also proven to be effective in treating the depression and anxiety disorders that often accompany Asperger Syndrome.

Difficulties

Although generally very useful, those with an Autism Spectrum Disorder may have a particularly difficult time with CBT. Most patients only go once or twice a week for an hour at a time for a set duration. Other patients may have to go more often or for longer because it is more difficult for them to communicate and identify emotions.

But this should not be a point of discouragement. Despite occasional setbacks and slower progress, CBT helps those with Asperger Syndrome with their lives in general. It is a holistic treatment that targets many symptoms at once, unlike many medications and other forms of therapy.

CBT is a vital part of living with Asperger Syndrome and other forms of autism. It can help reduce reliance on medication and improve the overall happiness of those with Asperger Syndrome-two huge achievements. But most importantly, the exercises and coping mechanisms learned in CBT are indispensable tools that can be used every day.

## TREATMENT FOR ASPERGER SYNDROME

Asperger syndrome is a neurobiological condition that affects children and adults. Many people feel it is a form of high functioning autism and it falls in the group of conditions of spectrum disorder or pervasive personality disorder. It affects the ability of the person to socialize and communicate effectively with others. Individuals often exhibit social communication, social interaction, and social imagination.

At this time doctors and researchers have not found a cause or cure for Asperger syndrome. There has been some research to indicate that individuals who suffer from this condition have had permanent changes to their frontal lobe. These changes make a difference in the ability of the brain to process social activities.

In 1944 Hans Asperger labeled this disorder autistic psychopathy and published a paper describing the symptoms and behaviors. However, it wasn't until 1994 that the disability was recognized in the DSM-IV. Throughout those years, and the many different research studies which have been performed, the exact cause of this disorder has never been found.

While there is currently no cure for Asperger syndrome there are treatment protocols that help both adults and children to learn how to interact more successfully in social situations.

Treatment which may be recommended will depend upon the individual's level of adaptive functioning. Just as with autism, there is a range of disability or functionality of individuals who have Asperger's.

Resources that are available for children and adults with Asperger syndrome are communication and social skills training which help individuals to learn the unwritten rules of socialization and communication. These are often too difficult for children in much the same way that students learn to speak a foreign language. This is because for children and adults with Asperger syndrome learning these social communication skills is a foreign language.

It is possible for children with Asperger syndrome to learn how to speak using a more natural rhythm as well as how to interpret communication such as gestures, eye contact, tone of voice, humor and sarcasm which usually fly right over the top of their heads.

Another behavioral therapy that may be recommended is cognitive behavior therapy. This technique is aimed at its decreasing problem behaviors such as interrupting, obsessions and angry outbursts. They also focused on helping children and adults to recognize a troubled situation, such as a new place or events, and then be able to select a specific strategy to cope.

While there is no medication specifically aimed at treatment of Asperger syndrome there are some symptoms that can be controlled, such as anxiety, depression or hyperactivity using medications. Most commonly, selective serotonin reuptake inhibitors, antipsychotics, and some stimulants are used to treat these problems.

Treatment outlook for individuals with Asperger syndrome is usually heavily correlated with the measured IQ. Those who have a high IQ will fare better and show greater improvements in social function than those who have a below average IQ.

Children who experience the symptoms of Asperger syndrome will also require a bit of assistance in the school system.

Schools that have a communications specialist with an interest in social skills training, opportunities for social interaction and structured settings, a concern for teaching real-life skills and a willingness to individualize the curriculum are best suited to help individuals who have Asperger syndrome. Parents should stay informed of what is happening in the child's classroom and maintain fre?uent communication with the teacher.

Even though a specific pill is not available for treatment for Asperger syndrome, and there is no cure, individuals who have this condition have a degree of adaptability to the environment when they are taught coping strategies and have a good support system in their relationships.

## TREATMENT AVAILABLE FOR A CHILD WITH ASPERGER SYNDROME

Since a child with Asperger Syndrome shows patterns of behaviors and problems that differ widely from others, any typical treatment regimen or medication cannot be prescribed. However, there are several treatments that are proven to help a lot with the child's condition and his development. These include the following:

Parents Education And Training. The

parents, aside from being the first teachers are the primary guardians who can reinforce help to a child with Aspergers. It is crucial that they're educated properly with the nature of the kid's condition. Therefore, as a child's parent, you should undergo this type of training so you can even teach your child with Asperger self-help abilities. Learning these skills helps children achieve maximum independence.

Social Skills Training. Since a child with Aspergers is having difficulty interacting with other individuals, even with kids of his age, the child must undergo social skills training. As a child's parent, you could start this training by yourself; however, it's more advantageous on your part and your child if you ask for the guidance of an expert. Specialized training programs exist for the development of social skills intended for children with Aspergers.

Language Development Programs. Even

holding a normal conversation might be difficult for a child with Aspergers. While most individuals learn these skills by observing others, the people with Asperger's Syndrome might need personal coaching using specialized language development programs. For faster development, parents should contribute by teaching the kid to start a conversation in the most approachable manner. Body language and eye-contact are effective approaches which promote the connection between the parent and the kid.

Cognitive Behavioral Therapy. Psychological conditions such as Aspergers Syndrome in all ages might be treated utilizing this therapy.

This therapy applies approaches designed to modify the way a child thinks, feels and reacts to a situation. It targets the overall behavior of the child, especially the repetitive actions the child often does. A therapist has the capability to establish a connection between him and the child in a way that the child can feel comfortable and conditioned.

Tender Loving Care. Adults, especially the parents, play a significant role in the development of the kid with Aspergers by showing extensive care and love to this kid. Teachers, babysitters, the rest of the family members, close friends, and everyone else must get involved in the training and should sustain strong affection to the child for its faster development. Never let the child feel isolated to its environment. Instead, make the kid feel that it belongs wherever it gets involved with, especially at home and school. And in every action you make, do it with tender loving care.

## HOW IS ASPERGER'S SYNDROME DIAGNOSED?

If you suspect your child to have this condition, bringing him or her to a doctor is a good idea. The doctor will ask you a series of questions regarding your child's behavior. Your child will undergo a series of tests analyzing his ability to communicate, express, read and write. Intellectual, emotional and psychological evaluations may be done as well. The evaluation might be made by a number of doctors since Asperger's is a bit hard to diagnose. Some may even mistake it for other developmental problems such as attention deficit/hyperactivity disorder or ADHD.

## HOW IS ASPERGER'S SYNDROME TREATED?

As mentioned earlier, there is no exact cure for Asperger's. The doctors will only recommend medications and therapies to lessen their severity and help the child cope and live to his optimum potential. There are no exact medications for Asperger's, but the doctor can prescribe drugs to relieve depression, anxiousness, and agitation which the child can manifest anytime. Therapies are also advised to improve the child's ability to communicate and understand people, and to improve his social skills. They are taught the right way of expressing how they feel and how to understand nonverbal cues such as eye contact, facial expressions, and other gestures. The child is also taught of ways to cope with certain situations such as going to school, meeting other people or transferring to another location.

## HOW CAN A PARENT HELP THE CHILD COPE?

Parents have the most important role in helping the child cope with this condition. They are the ones who have been with the child and are well-oriented about the situation.

You can learn about Asperger's. Education and information are very important in order to understand what your child is going through. You can ask your doctor, read medical books or journals, and research over the internet about the condition of your child. You can also read ways on how to cope with your child, especially during hard times.

Be familiar with your child's behavior. Not all children with Asperger's manifest the same symptoms and characteristics. By being familiar with your child's behavior, you also learn how to deal with it. Just have patience in going through tough times and show your child how supportive you can be.

Be active in therapies. Your child will undergo therapies until he or she is able to adjust. Be present in therapies so you can learn more about your child and his or her condition. Talk to the professionals in charge of the sessions so that you can also become part of the team.

Inform people about your child's condition.

Some parents may be hesitant about telling people about their child, but it is important to let others know about it. Inform the school, teachers, and people in your neighborhood about your child's condition so they can also adjust to your child.

Since children with Asperger's may have awkward social skills, others may misinterpret this and be judgmental if they are not properly informed.

# CHAPTER NINE
# ALTERNATIVE THERAPIES AND TREATMENTS FOR ASPERGER

## HERBS AND NATURAL REMEDIES

If you have a child that has been diagnosed with Asperger's syndrome, you want to find the best treatments available. Aspergers cannot be cured however, because it is not a disease. Treatments for children with Aspergers are designed to help them function better in the areas the condition have affected them. Others have found the following treatments for Aspergers to be effective.

In a lot of instances, children affected by Aspergers require several different strategies and healing methods. While the accurate reason that Aspergers happens is a mystery, it does have an effect on how a person's brain works. For this reason, signals can from time to time be assisted from biofeedback. There are some inventive programs that imply some potential, which inform individuals with Aspergers how to change their brainwaves to assist in overcoming a variety of dilemmas.

While this kind of treatment for Aspergers is considered experimental and is not widely accepted, some researchers claim that it can be highly effective. Asperger's is not a disease and it's important that you and your child realize this and that it simply means a person's brain works differently. Evidence is starting to show that historic people such as Albert Einstein, Thomas Jefferson, Beethoven, and Mozart had Asperger's syndrome. By focusing on their strengths, people with this condition can do well in today's technological society. Of course, children with Aspergers do have challenges, and some face serious problems, but the point is to keep in mind that they can still be highly successful as well.

Some herbs and other natural remedies have been found to help treat Aspergers, as well. It is possible to use herbal remedies to help calm a child with Aspergers down, help them focus, and to help reduce their anxiety.

For symptoms ranging from anxiety to depression, the supplement St. John's Wort can be used for both adults and children.

Passiflora also called passion flower, and chamomile is other herbal remedies that can be soothing to the nervous system. A homeopathic or herbal practitioner can give you more information on herbal remedies for treating specific symptoms of Aspergers.

Remember you are not alone as you face all the challenges that come with parenting a child with Aspergers. This condition is quite common, and fortunately, while there's no known cure, there are many ways to effectively deal with it. Some of the treatments discussed above may be of help to you and your family and make it a little easier to understand Asperger's syndrome.

## USING HERBS AND NATURAL PRODUCTS TO TREAT ASPERGERS

When it comes to medicating children afflicted with Asperger's syndrome, you will probably need to be both tolerant and inventive, as all children are a bit different and you might need to try a variety of strategies prior to recognizing the ones that work optimally. While you should meet with a qualified physician, psychologists, and school administrators, bear in mind that you know your child better than anyone else, therefore you should also put your acumen and talent for cognizance to use. The following are some remedies for Aspergers that may work excellently for your child.

Changes to routine are especially hard for children with Aspergers to handle, therefore stability is very important.

Assigning times for even simple tasks like free time, homework and mealtime will help give them structure in their routine. When choosing parenting styles many parents prefer to give their children more freedom, while others prefer this more rigid style. No matter what your preference is when it comes to kids with Aspergers, you aren't doing them a favor by giving them too much flexibility in such areas, as it will only confuse them.

You will lower their stress level when they know there is a routine that will be followed. Asperger's syndrome cannot be treated by one specific medication. The symptoms that come with this condition can be treated with medications, however. Many children with Aspergers also suffer from other conditions that can include ADD, bipolar disorder, and depression. Controlling these symptoms can be managed in some cases with medication. Any medication has to be tailored to the individual because Aspergers has such a wide range of symptoms. So, Aspergers can't be treated with a single drug but there are medications available to help with the various symptoms.

Some herbs and other natural remedies have been found to help treat Aspergers, as well. Depending on the particular problems the child has, certain herbal and homeopathic supplements may help them to calm down, focus or reduce their anxiety. The supplement St. John's Wort is used in adults and children to help with symptoms that range from anxiety to depression.

Passiflora also called passion flower, and chamomile is other herbal remedies that can be soothing to the nervous system. For additional information regarding herbal remedies that can be used to treat symptoms of Asperger's, talk to a homeopathic or herbal practitioner.

You can do many things to help a child with

Aspergers, and the specific approach you take has to be based on the child's unique needs. Under many circumstances, you can seek efficient treatments to aid with the tougher signs. While your child will always be a little different, there's no reason why he or she can't also lead a happy and productive life. The medications we've been researching for Aspergers can aid you in coming across the most excellent opportunities.

# CHAPTER TEN
# HOW ASPERGER SYNDROME CAUSES HARM TO ONE'S LIFE?

Many people might ask what Asperger syndrome is. Some may have heard of the name and thinking that they know something about it. In fact, the truth is, people are often unclear about the real meaning of it.

This illness has become more and more popular nowadays, commonly well known over the past twenty years. Some writers have already written about it and released the books. They are either position of people who have been diagnosed with it or the people who have the responsibility to take care of them. Most of the books out in the market are mentioning the effects of Asperger syndrome in children, trying to suggest ways to help and manage them. It can be of great help to be able to spot children with Asperger syndrome in the earlier stage. This can be extremely helpful to both the parents and the child, even though resources are still limited.

Despite the limited resources, the increased rate of diagnosis does tend to mean that at least the child's problems are recognized early, much better for the people around them. Social functioning and education are specially arranged and supported this type of children.

Last time, Asperger syndrome was not well known, hence this type of specialist support are unlikely to be available. However, there are still the majority of the adults out there who have Asperger syndrome but has never been diagnosed, or even received their diagnosis up till now. They will most probably experience problems like struggling through their childhood or adolescence days feeling alienated and misunderstood. For those people around them, they will feel perplexed and frustrated. The difficulties could have been perhaps, minimized if the condition is recognized much earlier are more likely to become entrenched problems.

If you are the one with this condition and just received a diagnosis, or even someone you help is down with it, you can understand more about Asperger syndrome and its irrational behavior. There are also suggesting avenues to look into if you wish to verify a diagnosis.

For adults with Asperger syndrome, they are always appeared to be eccentric or odd to others. A few of the less fortunate may have been wrongly diagnosed with other conditions. In fact, many of them will still be struggling there miserably. This article aims to describe the different kinds of difficulties people encountered and experienced, also to suggest methods for the people around them to be able to help. It also aims to help people who are struggling to support individuals with Asperger syndrome to find other ways of handling. Do not forget, they may be one of your close ones, be it family member, partner or friends.

## THE IMPORTANCE OF TESTING FOR ASPERGER SYNDROME

Asperger syndrome is on the mild end of spectrum disorders or pervasive personality disorders. Because of the characteristics and criteria for the diagnosis of Asperger syndrome it is related to autism. Many times it has been considered a silent disability because it was only after 1994 when it was recognized in the DSM-IV and even later than that before professionals and parents recognized the condition.

Some consider Asperger syndrome a developmental condition because the majority of individuals have normal intelligence and normal language development, but what falls short is social interaction. At this time there is no one specific conclusive diagnostic tests used to determine if an individual has Asperger syndrome. Instead, diagnosis and testing is done between the physician, a child's teacher and parents. At times, a psychologist is brought into the picture to evaluate peer relationships, reactions to new situations and the ability to understand feelings or other types of indirect communication.

In an effort to increase the social awareness of individuals who suffer from Asperger syndrome, and therefore the acceptance of these individuals, there has been some development of individual's tasks which help to point sufferers in the direction of a potential diagnosis. While these tests are often found online, they may not be completely accurate.

However, they do help to point individuals in the direction needed in order to find how for their social situation.

These online tests are more accurate in adult situations than they are in the pediatric population. In other words, most of them are designed to ask questions which relate to adult activities and not to those experienced in the classroom. Children are best served by an evaluation with their primary care practitioner, psychologist and with the assistance of their parents.

Growing up with this disorder leaves children at higher risk to bullies and cruel teasing by their peers.

Children are more at risk because those

with Asperger syndrome will find that they are unable to interact socially with their peers in the way that their classmates are capable of. Individuals with Asperger's often have difficulty with social communication, social interaction, and social imagination. This basically means that, although these children have normal or above average intelligence and normal language development, they are often unable to participate in social interaction with their peers which sets them apart for teasing.

One Asperger syndrome quiz that may help individuals to determine their risk factor for this diagnosis can be found online.

Adults who suffer from Asperger syndrome find they are never really able to grasp conversations that involve small talk and would rather sit with the computer than with adults.

When adults approach their doctor for

diagnosis the testing usually starts with an IQ test.

Doctors may also administer autism diagnostic observation schedule for high-functioning verbal young adults. Both tests allow a doctor to look at social communication skills and behavior.

DEPRESSION AND ASPERGER SYNDROME

Depression is often comorbid with Asperger Syndrome, meaning it isn't a side effect or symptom but rather an entirely separate condition that accompanies it. It is very common for those with some form of autism to also be diagnosed with depression. Studies have shown that more high-functioning forms, like Asperger Syndrome, show the greatest prevalence.

Feelings of isolation, an inability to recognize emotions in oneself and others, and difficulties operating in a social world are common in those with Asperger

Syndrome, and can easily lead to depression. Some believe that the changes autism causes in the brain may make those with the condition naturally more susceptible. The reason may be environmental, or chemical, or both.

Depression can exacerbate some of the worst symptoms associated with Asperger Syndrome, like self-harm and obsession. Plus, the overlap in symptoms, like social withdrawal and impaired communication can make it difficult to diagnose. Teens, particularly those in late adolescence, are especially susceptible. You can see why it's such a serious problem.

Treatment for depression usually involves some form of talk therapy. This itself presents some difficulties, although many have seen results. Because those who have Autism Spectrum Disorders have trouble identifying their feelings and communicating with others, therapy sessions may take longer than usual. Instead, CBT is often used to help treat thought patterns and specific circumstances and situations that may trigger depression and other symptoms. Current research has focused on finding particular methods for specifically helping autistic patients.

Medication has shown to be slightly more effective, although it, too, is highly controversial. Antipsychotics like Ability have been proven to treat symptoms of depression and Asperger Symptom and have been approved by the FDA for both. But side effects, dosage, and a long transition period turn many off of medication.

The good news is that major steps are being taken to solve this problem. Spreading awareness about the prevalence of depression is a top priority in the autism community. Researchers from psychiatry and pharmacology are working on understanding the link between the two and developing a more effective way to treat them at the same time. Recognizing the problem is half the battle. Educating parents and partners on what to look out for can ensure that those with Asperger Syndrome and other forms of autism can begin to get the help they need.

# CHAPTER ELEVEN
# THE RANGE OF DISABILITY WITH ASPERGERS SYNDROME

Asperger's syndrome is considered one of the disabilities included in the autism spectrum disorders or personality pervasive disorders. Often times it is classified as a high functioning form of autism because these sufferers will have normal or above average intelligence and normal language development.

Individuals who suffer from Asperger's syndrome will have more difficulty with communicating with others and have a triad of symptoms which include poor social imagination, poor social interaction and poor social communication. In many cases, they are unable to maintain eye contact and do not read and react to social cues that most of us do subconsciously.

Some question whether or not Asperger's

syndrome is truly a disability but should rather be termed a difference in ability.

The fact is, a great number of individuals who suffer from the symptoms also have special abilities that can't be ignored. These abilities often fall into the realm of math or music. This should not be confused with the individual who has autism, but a highly developed skill or talent and considered a savant.

The difference lies in the individual's language development and intelligence level. Individuals with Aspergers can have a chance to become very productive functioning people in society if the right steps are taken to help them develop strategies and coping mechanisms to attempt to overcome their symptoms.

The symptoms and condition of Asperger's syndrome have no known cure. At this time researchers believe that it is the result of a neurological deficit in the brain which manifests itself as a difficulty in social interactions. Because the functioning and structure of the brain cannot be changed individuals must learn to develop coping strategies that will help them interact with society and decrease their frustration level.

The range of abilities and disabilities of individuals who have Asperger's syndrome is very wide. There are some who have the same behavioral issues that face those who have autism while others appear to be quite at ease in social situations and exhibited only some mild obsessive-compulsive disorders or ritualistic behavior. Frustration sets in for both the individual and their family members when the sufferer may refuse to seek any kind of help because of a lack of being able to see the future and have any hope for the future.

A diagnosis of Asperger's syndrome in childhood often occurs after the age of three while autism is usually diagnosed prior to the age of three. There is no guarantee of the future for those who suffer the symptoms of Asperger's syndrome but it has been found that individual counseling to help people develop coping strategies and family counseling to help family members cope with behaviors that are not intentional is the best answer to increasing the ability of an individual to function in society.

Family members and parents often have questions about what the future will hold for their child and sibling after the diagnosis of Asperger's syndrome. Unfortunately, physicians and psychologists are on able to give an accurate picture of what the future will look like because of the wide range of disability that an individual may experience throughout their lifetime. All that can be assured is that their family member can now receive care and treatment that was not available prior to 1994 when the diagnosis was first entered into the DSM-IV.

Although it is a small consolation, research continues to delve into causes and treatments that can help those individuals who have Asperger's syndrome or high functioning autism.

# CHAPTER TWELVE
# ASPERGER'S SYNDROME
# AT WORK

If you are like many people with Asperger's Syndrome, you categorize small talk as a nonsensical NT (neurotypical) ritual where people waste time talking about stupid subjects that no one really cares about.

However, small talk is actually a critical workplace skill. It is the first step in establishing those all-important relationships with your colleagues. Most neurotypicals (who make up the majority of the workforce) place a high value on relationships. So much so that a good relationship with one's supervisor and liking one's co-workers are consistently rated as major factors for job satisfaction.

Sharing a few friendly comments with fellow employees you see in the lunchroom or in the elevator sends the message that you consider yourself to be part of the group. Small talk with your workmates is the starting point for building camaraderie and trust.

You do not need to actually like someone in order to act friendly with them at work. Sometimes small actions go a long way toward establishing yourself as likable. For example:

Greet co-workers you see or interact with in the morning by saying "Good morning" or asking "Hi, how are you?"

Smile when you greet people or pass them in the hallway. If necessary, practice so that it becomes natural. A person who doesn't smile is often perceived as angry or aloof.

Join your colleagues for lunch on a regular basis.

How to Make Small Talk?

Small talk is the discussion of general, neutral topics for short periods of time (usually no more than 5 minutes). Neutral topics are things like the weather, traffic, sports, a national news item, plans for the weekend, etc. Topics to avoid are those that polarize people (politics, religion, race), make them feel uncomfortable (sexual topics), or personal observations (weight, clothing, hairstyle, mannerisms). Negative comments about other employees or the company should also be avoided.

If you do not follow sports teams or popular programs on television, you can still find subjects for small talk. Many local news stations have Web sites that provide brief summaries of top stories. This is a quick way to stay informed about what is happening in your community. The point of small talk is making connections with others. To do this, you must keep a discussion going for at least two or three turns. If you reply to a question or comment with a one-word answer or by saying "I don't know," it won't go any farther.

Let's say you are in the break room and someone asks whether you saw a particular program or sports event. You answer, "No." Oops! The conversation is over. Instead ask a question to express your interest in the other person, such as, "I haven't seen that program, what is it about?" or "I don't follow baseball. Do you play?"

Here is another example that illustrates how small talk can be the bridge for establishing good relationships with your co-workers. Someone asks, "Did you get caught in that traffic jam on Route 66?" Instead of saying "no," you say, "No, I live in Smithtown so I don't take the highway to get here." The other person responds, "I used to drive through Smithtown when I worked at ACME Widget works." You reply, "I worked at ACME six years ago in the R&D group." Your new acquaintance says, "I was in R&D, too. We should get together for lunch this week."

This kind of scenario is not uncommon and can be the start of productive, long-term business relationships. Even though it may feel uncomfortable for you at first, look at small talk as an important business skill to practice.

## PRACTICAL TIPS TO HELP YOUR EMPLOYEE WITH ASPERGER SYNDROME GET ESTABLISHED IN YOUR OFFICE

You have just hired someone who has Asperger Syndrome, or perhaps you suspect so, and indeed he or she has very strong skills to match the job description. It is likely that you will be very pleased because people with Asperger Syndrome tend to have a strong focus and commitment to a job well done.

To set up for office place success, you will find it pays off to invest in some training time, early on in some of those skills unrelated to the primary job, but fundamentally important to navigating the day at the office.

Here are seven straightforward strategies to help your new employee prosper and produce for your business.

1. Logical lists. As you see a routine or task that requires daily attention, log it on a list. Explaining the purpose behind the task may help it to become automatic.

People with Asperger Syndrome like to make sense out of things.

2. Create a 'cheat sheet' for phone coverage. If you want your employee to pinch hit on the phones, have a few generic phrases that work for your workplace, for example, "Can I have someone get back to you with that information?"

3. Be very specific about what you expect in general office matters. Help her to know where more and less flexibility is in order and appropriate in the daily flow of the workplace. What routines must be done one way only? Observe, make notes and plan for periodic feedback time.

4. Be prepared to give your input with some of the smaller steps you may not typically think of stating. Gradually transfer responsibility and accountability to your employee, withdrawing your level of involvement as you see him catching on to the rhythms of your office place.

5. Help her become comfortable with the social culture of your workplace. People with Asperger tend to want to stay focused on tasks they enjoy. Being specific about when to go for breaks and lunch will be a guide for opportunities to personally connect with co-workers.

6. Have a set routine for evaluation and

feedback sessions. Start the meeting by talking about the qualities you see in your new employee. "Here's where your work is very well done." Be sensitive to feelings of past failure with social and organizational issues. Your employee with Asperger is probably quite familiar with his weaknesses, having heard about them and struggled with them in some other past setting. You can say " Here's where we will work together:"

7. Don't be afraid to be blunt. It will be helpful. There is a distinction between 'blunt' and 'rude.' He will appreciate and understand directness and clarity. If you are finding yourself repeating requests, you can say, "What plan can we come up with to help you establish routines that I have been reminding you about?"

## SOCIAL SKILLS IN THE WORKPLACE

## TRUE LIFE STORY

We again visit the workplace of employer 'Jack' and his new employee 'Al' who has Asperger Syndrome. In this small informal office, Al felt discomfort and confusion with ordinary routines related to phones, break time and workplace jargon. In this next phase of our work together, we designed three customized action plans, which helped Al succeed with the more social side of office responsibilities.

Jack: "When it comes to the job he was hired to do, Al is outstanding. But when people skills are required, he flounders. He goes off topic or seems confused about what people do in ordinary daily situations."

Jack decided he would work directly and discreetly with Al, to help him feel less 'centered out' for this personalized training program. Co-workers had 'supporting roles' but Jack was the one-to-one trainer and advocate for Al. We created action plans for these three social aspects of office life:

1. Telephone Conversation Skills

2. Flexibility and Feelings of Fitting In

3. Expressions of Speech

Goal 1 Telephone conversation skills

Jack: "Sometimes we have to rely on Al to cover phones for parts of the day when the office is short on staff. Al tells me he has had some bad experiences trying to figure out what to say on the phone. I can see he is anxious about this."

The Plan: Al and Jack created a phone answering 'script sheet' that gave Al the words and phrases for opening greetings, message taking, transferring calls, general comments about who to speak to for what, and a few social niceties.

The role-played privately in Jack's office. Jack asked Al to keep his conversations business-like brief. Al's scripted answer to

"How are you today?" was "Fine, thank you." since Al was sometimes tempted to answer with enthusiastic details more appropriate for a social conversation with friends. If someone's question threw him a curve, Al's SOS script was "Please hold for someone who can help you." and immediately transfer the call to Jack or Jack's assistant. Al's phone skills grew and on his own initiative, he spent time sitting in areas where he could listen and learn from co-workers fielding phone calls.

Goal 2 Flexibility and feelings of fitting in

Jack: "Al gets fixated on his work. It's a quality that turns into a disadvantage at times. Other things come with this job! Time is open-ended for Al! I want him to know when to focus on something else that needs to be taken care of, or even just have lunch."

The Plan: This was a two-step plan:

1. Jack worked with Al to clarify and prioritize tasks that could be done over time, and tasks that had deadlines that were more pressing. He explained to Al that it was important and encouraged to stop and take breaks on occasions that threw the usual routine off schedule, such as an office staff meeting or a birthday gathering.

2. Jack and Al collaborated on a set of guiding questions, which helped to steer Al into another activity, if necessary. To help him break focus and evaluate, Al set his watch to beep three times a day to remind him to review his questions list:

"Is there something else I need to tend to right now?"

"Is something going on that everyone else is a part of?"

"What do I need to do before getting back to my work?"

Al faithfully relied on his 'guiding ?uestions' once he experienced how good it felt to fit in with the normal office rhythms.

Goal 3 Expressions of speech

Office life had its own culture and early on Al was grappling with language that, for him, was a garble of confusing messages.

Jack: "Al is really mystified by phrases we all take for granted here. When we use expressions new to Al, like 'shift gears' or 'hit the ground running' I can see he is baffled. When a co-worker said "I am fit to be tied," Al did not make the connection that his co-worker was feeling short of patience and frustrated.

The Plan: Al was encouraged to be honest and ask people to rephrase statements or instructions he did not understand. One of Al's strengths was a memory for information so once he understood he was on board when the expression came up again. His co-workers were very kind in helping him with work-place vocabulary and Al enjoyed that support.

It was thrilling for him to experience the feeling of belonging in this office, so it got to be something of a game for Al to find new work-related figures of speech.

These action plans took time and planning but were successful because Jack saw the long-term value in the commitment required. And Al, who was painfully aware of his social skill 'deficits' was receptive to the program and delighted with the good feelings that come with support and progress.


## DIAGNOSIS AND STRATEGIES FOR MARRIAGE WITH ASPERGER'S SYNDROME

Neurological differences like Asperger

Syndrome can be seen as necessary evolutionary adaptations rather than pathologies. An alternate mindset rather than a disorder. The following strategies can be useful:

1. Pursuing a Diagnosis: A diagnosis can be important to acknowledge ASD traits that might be causing marital problems; however, it is not required to apply these strategies. Understanding how ASD traits affect the relationship can remove the blame, frustration, shame, pain and confusion felt by one or both partners. A diagnosis can be obtained from a clinician skilled in identifying adult ASD. They must also have a thorough understanding of the neurodiverse dynamic. It is especially helpful if the evaluation includes an interview with the spouse.

2. Accepting the ASD diagnosis

While evaluating the relationship in light of the diagnosis and accepting it, seeking information is key. An ASD-specific couple's counselor and Spouse-and-Couples-Support Groups can be really helpful. Individuals with ASD can be loyal, honest, intelligent, hardworking, generous, and funny. Accepting their strengths and weakness can lead to a more balanced picture of the marriage.

### 3. Staying motivated

Sometimes the NS partner may be so depressed, angry, and completely disconnected from her partner, that she might not desire to salvage the marriage. It is always helpful when both partners are motivated to address and change the issues in their marriage.

### 4. Understanding how ASD impacts the individual

Understanding that ASD is a biologically-based, neurological difference vs. a psychological mental disorder is key. Psychoeducation is an important part of sorting out the challenges in ASD marriages. Books, movies, and workshops can help both partners better understand ASD. They can then implement ASD-specific strategies in their relationship. Due to its complex nature, learning about ASD is lifelong.

## 5. Managing depression, anxiety, OCD, and ADHD

People with ASD are at increased risk for depression, anxiety, obsessive-compulsive disorder (OCD), or attention deficit hyperactivity disorder (ADHD). It is vital to diagnose and treat these mental health issues with medications and therapy. Untreated they can have serious negative conse uences for both partners. NS spouses can often experience their own mental health issues such as anxiety, depression, Affective Deprivation Disorder, and Post-Traumatic Stress Disorder (PTSD), as a result of being in a relationship with an undiagnosed ASD partner. In these cases, the NS partner should also receive treatment.

6. Self-Awareness for the NS partner

The NS partner can often be a super nurturer and manager. She may have also have her own issues, and sometimes even ASD traits, and other neurological differences such as ADHD, dyslexia, mood and anxiety disorders. Self-awareness for the NS spouse can also help her understand why she chose her partner with ASD, the part she plays in the conflicts with her partner, and what she can do about it.

7. Creating a relationship schedule

A calendar is an important tool for any marriage. Due to the executive functioning and social-emotional reciprocity problems that adults with ASD have, keeping a calendar is even more crucial in a neurodiverse marriage. Additionally, a relationship schedule can help the couple plan for conversation, sex, and leisure activities in order to stay connected.

## 8. Meeting each other's sexual needs

The partner with ASD tends to either want a lot of sexual activity or too little. Scheduling sex to accommodate the needs of both spouses can help regulate their sex-life. The partner with ASD may also be mechanical and unemotional in bed, or he may struggle with sex due to sensory sensitivities. The partner with ASD may need to be taught how to maintain a daily emotional connection-both inside and outside the bedroom.

## 9. Bridging parallel play

A partner with ASD may go days, weeks, or even months engrossed in his own special interest, and not spend time with his partner. This "parallel play" can leave his partner feeling lonely and abandoned. Common activities that might have brought the couple together whilst dating can abruptly stop after marriage. This is in part due to his challenges in initiation, reciprocity, planning, and organizing. Scheduling playing together-long walks, boat rides, hikes, and travel can help bridge the parallel play gap.

## 10. Coping with sensory overload and stress

Sensory sensitivity is a core trait of ASD. A person's senses may be either hypersensitive or hypersensitive (diminished sensitivity): a caress can feel like burning fire, or a needle prick can have no effect. Strategies can help prevent meltdowns triggered by a sensory overload. Individuals with ASD can also be more susceptible to stress than their non-autistic counterparts. Planning time to self-care and relax is crucial.

## 11. Developing theory of mind (TOM)

The partner with ASD tends to have a weak TOM-he may have trouble understanding, predicting and responding to a person's thought-feeling state. He may unintentionally say and do things that can come across as insensitive and hurtful to his partner. He can develop a better TOM by becoming more aware, of how he is likely to offend his partner. He may also be able to express more complimentary and affirmative speech.

## 12. Improving communication

A core feature of ASD is communication challenges. The partner with ASD might have difficulties in picking up facial cues, vocal intonations, and body language. He can often monopolize, or have difficulty initiating conversations, and keeping them flowing. His partner might feel frustrated by the lack of communication and reciprocity.

Scheduling daily conversation time, and direct communication strategies can be useful.

13. Co-parenting strategies

Individuals with ASD can be very good parents when it comes to concrete tasks, such as helping children with homework, teaching them certain skills, or taking them on outdoor adventures. In order to meet his children's emotional needs, he might need cues from his NS partner. Working with a parenting coach can also prove valuable.

14. Managing expectations and assuming the positive

Adjusting expectations based on ability and neurology is important for both partners. Working hard to improve the marriage with the strategies listed here can bring about real change. Resetting entrenched patterns of interaction can often be challenging. Personal growth can often be arduous and slow; however, both partners must assume the positive of each other.

## 15. Couples counseling for neurodiverse marriage

Neurodiverse couples report that working with a counselor, unfamiliar with ASD harmed their relationship. An ASD-specific couple's counselor can teach both partners about ASD, and interpret the neurodiverse points of view. Counseling can help a couple brainstorm and implement strategies to better their relationship.

The issues and challenges that some neurodiverse couples face can seem similar, but every individual with ASD is unique. Couples have to solve their marital challenges in a manner that is best suited to their situation and needs.

## ASPERGER'S SYNDROME CONCERNS

Asperger's syndrome (AS) or Asperger's disorder (AD) is a pervasive developmental disorder characterized by a conjuncture of symptoms such as qualitative impairment of social interaction, repetitive or stereotypical behavior, activities, and interests, physical clumsiness. To be noted that unlike autism, Asperger's does not affect the normal cognitive and language development of the patient.

Currently, there are several screening instruments used by pediatricians or general practitioners to diagnose a child suffering from Asperger's as soon as he/she is 30 months old. Some of these screening instruments are Asperger Syndrome Diagnostic Scale, Childhood Asperger Syndrome Test, Gilliam Asperger's Disorder Scale, Autism Spectrum Quotient, Krug Asperger's Disorder Index, and Autism

Spectrum Screening Questionnaire.

The exact causes of Asperger's syndrome are not known, however, there is enough evidence to suggest a genetic contribution. It seems that AS runs in the family, although no specific gene has been linked to the disorder. Apparently, the likelihood for a child to be born with AS increases with every family member who manifests behavioral symptoms such as difficulties with exposure and management of social interactions and/or problems with reading or language. Other theories suggest that AS can result from prenatal exposure to agents that cause birth defects.

The first symptom of children suffering from AS is impaired social interaction. Specifically, their social behavior has been characterized as "active but odd". While people with AS may cognitively understand the concept of emotion or empathy, being able to theorize and accept them as facts, they will still not be able to show them in a social context. As a result, they might come off as rude, insensitive, indifferent or annoying, although willing to engage and talk. Some children manifest what is known as "selective mutism" when they will speak only to the individuals they like or want to while remaining perfectly silent in the presence of others.

By the age of 5 or 6, a child suffering from AS will start displaying an unusually focused interest in some activity or field of knowledge, easily memorizing detailed information or data about a narrow subject.

This amazing display of memory capacity is counteracted by the fact that he/she is not able to see the bigger picture or the context of the information held. Although an AS child's interests can vary with time, he/she will still be immersed into pursuing one specific and narrow part of a subject. Also, other more or less complex body movements become highly stereotyped (flapping, clapping, head turning, pirouette, etc.).

With regard to language and speech development, although no clinical delays have been reported, the acquisition and use of language is rather atypical. For example, a child with AS cannot understand a joke, a fantasy story, metaphors or figurative language in general because he/she interprets them literally.

# CHAPTER THIRTEEN
# ASPERGERS TREATMENT OPTIONS

An overview on the Aspergers treatment will give you an idea on how to deal with this syndrome. Anyone can suffer from this disorder although experts believe that a great percentage involves children. Parenting can be tough if you have a child with this condition or autism. The treatment will depend on the severity of the disorder and in most cases, it involves medication.

Symptomatic treatment is used for Aspergers Syndrome. This means that the medical professional will consider the symptoms that are exhibited by the patient and the damage that the person has suffered from. The symptom will vary from one person to another and so you must seek expert advice before using any type of treatment. When you see the common symptoms of this condition, you have to visit the doctor right away.

Most of the treatments are geared towards helping the patient live a normal life. There is no sense in making the patient too dependent. The patient needs rehabilitation wherein he or she will learn the ways to live a more independent lifestyle. This is possible if the parents and family are willing to cooperate. Aside from this, medical professionals can also recommend social skills training, behavioral modification, parent education, psychotherapy, and many others. Psychopharmacological and psychosocial interventions are necessary. In some situations, medications and educational interventions are also necessary. This may include the use of tricyclic antidepressants, neuroleptics, beta blockers, mood stabilizers, and psychostimulants.

The Aspergers Syndrome has core

symptoms which include physical clumsiness, repetitive or obsessive routines, and poor communication capability. The right Aspergers treatment is necessary and this should be introduced on the onset of the symptoms. Parents should be watchful of these symptoms because if you ignore it, you will have greater problems over time. When the condition is addressed at an earlier date, the patient can learn to properly interact with others. Some patients are able to communicate well with their families and friends.

If you want your child to be self-sufficient and function effectively at home or in school, you have to act now. You must work closely with an expert in this type of condition so that the right Aspergers treatment can be identified. In some cases, this can be a trial and error method because some treatments might not work. Different methods can be used until the right one is found. This can be a lengthy process but with patience and determination, families can succeed.

Hyperactive, impulsive, and inattentive patients are harder to deal with and so psychostimulants can be given but with doctor's prescription. The patient can be given metamphetamine, dextroamphetamine, and methyphenidate.

Mood stabilizers are usually given to patients that show aggression and irritability. This can include lithium, carbamazepine, and valproate. Children with anxieties may be given tri-cyclic antidepressants such as nortriptyline, clomipramine, and imipramine, as well as SSRIs. These are some of the treatments available for Aspergers Syndrome. You can also find natural treatments out there but you have to work it out with your doctor. This is a serious condition that you must deal with properly.

## FAMOUS PEOPLE WITH ASPERGER'S SYNDROME

Recently, some researchers suggested that such well-known personalities from the past, like Albert Einstein and Isaac Newton had Asperger's syndrome. Scientists say that they showed some tendencies of the syndrome in their behavior, such as an intense interest in one topic, or social problems. Naturally, the absence of diagnosis during life does not mean that there was nothing to diagnose, especially if we bear in mind that while there was no widespread knowledge about the syndrome (as often happens with Asperger's syndrome, which recently has been widely recognized in psychiatric circles). However, such a post-mortem diagnosis remains controversial.

Arguments in favor of the alleged autism spectrum disorders infamous personalities vary from person to person. Some of them argue that in the case of Albert Einstein (one of the most freꞯuently cited suspected autistic), he learned to talk late, was a lonely kid, organized violent tantrums, silently repeated the previously pronounced sentence, and needed his wives to play the role of parents when he was an adult - the stereotypical factors for autistic individuals.

Isaac Newton stuttered and suffered from epilepsy. Many of these alleged historical cases of Asperger's syndrome can be ꞯuite soft (not expressed), but some skeptics argue that in these cases only some features of autism can be seen, and they are not enough to diagnose autism spectrum. In the end, many critics of historical diagnosis claim that it is simply impossible to diagnose the dead, and therefore nothing can be said with certainty about historic individuals with (or without) Asperger's syndrome.

All of these assumptions may be just an

attempt to create a pattern of behavior (role model, an object for imitation) for people with autism, and demonstrate that they can do constructive things, and make a contribution to society. Such a presumptive diagnosis is often used by activists for the rights of people with autism to show that the treatment of autism would be a loss to society. But others in the organizations for the rights of autistic people do not like these arguments because they feel that people with autism have to appreciate their uniꢀueness even if they do not want to be healed, regardless of whether people like Einstein were autistic.

Some features of appearance and facts of activity indicate that John Carmack is also a man with AS, or he has other unusual personality types of a similar nature. Possible causes and origins of Asperger's syndrome is hotly debated and controversial topic. The majority opinion today is that the causes of Asperger's syndrome are the same as autism's. Some researchers, however, disagree and argue that Asperger syndrome and autism are lead by two different things. All this occurs during the ongoing wider debate about whether Asperger's syndrome and other conditions (such as attention deficit disorder and hyperactivity disorder - ADHD) are the part of the so-called autism spectrum.

Among many competing theories about the causes of autism (and, therefore, as many believe to be Asperger's Syndrome.

## LIVING WITH ASPERGER'S SYNDROME

Ben did very well in the early grades learning to read and spell. His writing, however, was atrocious. He became a wonderful reader and seemed to comprehend everything he read. Also, he became an excellent speller and absorbed correct grammar and punctuation along the way.

His math skills seemed to be the weakest link in his learning process. In the early grades, he did fine in math, but in middle school and high school, math was definitely a problem for him.

In kindergarten, the children were playing "Duck, Duck, Goose." It is a game that requires the one who is "it" to choose another child to be the next "it." When he did not get chosen, he would cry and cry. We later learned this to be the beginning of a life filled with depression.

Some teachers learned that Ben would obey written commands better than oral instructions. During these elementary years was when we discovered there was a disconnect between what he heard and what his brain processed. Some, without realizing his disability, though he was lazy or just did not want to obey. Ben has always appeared so very normal; however, his disability was and is as real as one who cannot get around without a wheelchair.

When Ben was nine years old a psychologist from the Mayo Clinic in Minneapolis, Minnesota, came to South Dakota, where Ben and his family lived at the time. It was then that he was diagnosed with Asperger's Syndrome. The psychologist explained that the Asperger's Syndrome was like an umbrella under Autism and under it was also Attention Deficit Disorder, Obsessive Compulsive Disorder, and Depression (At least in Ben's case).

Shortly after the diagnosis, Ben's dad was transferred to Randolph Air Force Base, TX. and we began the process of learning all we could about the disorder. Ben's mom heard about a conference that was going to be held in the Dallas area. Dr. Tony Attwood, the leading expert in the field of Asperger Syndrome at the time, was to be the main speaker. She attended the conference and came away with a wealth of helpful information.

As an aside, when Ben heard that she was going to the conference, he said, "Good, Mom. Maybe you can learn how I can make friends." Ben had no friends and it was sad when his birthday came around because there was no one to invite to his birthday party. He realized this and was actually grieved because of it.

# CHAPTER FOURTEEN
# EDUCATIONAL SERVICES
# FOR ASPERGERS
# SYNDROME

Aspergers Syndrome is one of the conditions that belong to the autism spectrum of disorders. It is a broad spectrum of developmental delays, conditions, or disabilities that includes autism as one of its symptoms. Along with others, they belong to a spectrum of disorders because any of these symptoms could combine with other similar symptoms with autism.

This condition is generally uncommon; it is known to affect about four hundred thousand families in the United States alone. Although the diagnosis of this condition is generally difficult, it gets easier at an early age, typically about three years old. Treatment is similar to Autism with behavioral modifications and lots of therapy.

The number one characteristic that is typical of this condition is their poor social skills. They may show social interaction that is not typical of an average child--it may be inappropriate at times and also quite minimal. They may be able to communicate but in repetitive words and phrases, and their movements may be unusual. They tend to develop mannerisms and movements that are too awkward for a common child. They also lack cognitive skills such as reading, writing, and solving math problems, but most of these skills are combated when they go to a special needs school.

What makes them different from Autism is that these kids usually do not have any delays in language development, although they may have trouble using it in social context. There are also no obvious delays in activities of daily living.

These kids can bathe, eat, and dress like any other normal kid. They may even have higher intelligence than most kids of their age.

These kids can become the best that they can be with proper education and therapy. The symptoms may differ from one child to the next so they need to have the best care possible that is suited to their individual needs. This condition varies a lot so the choice of service is essential in determining which works best with your child.

As a parent, we all know dealing with a child with special needs is very challenging. Therefore we need all the help we can get to help them grow to be the best that they can be. Nurture their skills and capabilities through schools that offer techniques for children with special needs. They may need several sessions of physical therapy and occupational therapy to further promote their functional abilities.

Treatment for this condition may include a lot of specialized education intervention, training in social interaction, sensory integration, behavioral modification, and parent education. All these managements are being assisted by a professional that a parent needs to work with in order to bring out the best holistic approach.

## ENROLLING A TEENAGER WITH ASPERGERS SYNDROME AT A THERAPEUTIC SCHOOL

Aspergers syndrome is a disability that affects how a person relates to other people. People who have Aspergers may talk a lot about their hobbies but have problems in getting messages across other people or giving them a chance to talk. They may also have problems in understanding other people's feelings or their body gestures. Overall, it can be said that people with Aspergers have impaired communication with other people.

Aspergers is also demonstrated when people like their habits to be stringently observed and organized. They like everything to be at the right schedule and can be seriously frustrated when it is done in the "wrong" manner. The results of Aspergers vary and can range from formalized behavior to aggressive and anti-social behavior.

Secondary school can be highly upsetting for students with Aspergers syndrome given the secondary school's routine. Transferring classrooms and meeting new classmates and teachers can be extremely stressful for someone who likes everything to be "in place" or unchanging. A person who has Aspergers can also extend a lot of effort when speaking with others. While other students have better interpersonal relationship as they get older, people with Aspergers may find it tricky to maintain friendships.

A research by psychologist, investigates individuals with Aspergers from children between 14 and 18 years old. The thesis, which was based on interviews, self-evaluations and tests, found out that people afflicted with Aspergers were as comfortable as the comparison group. Although both Aspergers and comparison group established good relationships with their family, the former seems to have a difficult time building relationships outside the family sphere. With this, a therapeutic school can help people afflicted with Aspergers syndrome to gain more interpersonal skills, which permit them to relate with other people.

Hence, specialty schools such as an Aspergers school can help students get used to the school environment without much trauma. These schools have individualized programs that serve the needs of a person who struggles with a specific difficulty.

For example, people with Aspergers can work with groups, such as clubs, that permit them to polish their hobbies. Although they are fascinated about a specific subject and have a difficult time keeping up with other subjects, personalized programs can help these adolescents concentrate on subjects where they are performing poorly.

Adolescents dealing with Aspergers can also experience burnout in terms of school work. Thus, facing homework can be even more daunting when they do not have colleagues to share it with. Therapeutic schools can work out with teachers to modify schoolwork for these students without actually lowering coursework quality. A school counselor can also help these students in developing positive attitudes in dealing with their interpersonal difficulties.

## SHOULD CHILDREN WITH AUTISM OR ASPERGERS SYNDROME BE SUSPENDED FROM SCHOOL?

Should children with Autism or Aspergers Syndrome (or other related disorders) be suspended from school? If the child is in a regular public/private school and is overly aggressive toward other students or teachers, what to do? What if they are on an IEP at this school?

If the child is attending a special school due to their condition, does it make sense that the child be suspended? What about the age of the child? Should a child of 5 or 8 years old be suspended? What about a child of 12 or 13? Any difference if the child is 16 with a disorder?

Certainly if the child is on an IEP that recognizes their disorder or they are attending a special school that claims to be able to help children with the child's disorder, then NO, they should NOT suspend the child. Age MAY play a role in certain cases.

That said, it is important to recognize every child is different. When it comes to these disorders, they are all different and two children with the same exact disorders, same age, similar backgrounds can have very different views and understanding of the world around them. It might be appropriate to suspend one child, but the other may simply not fully understand the seriousness. The point simply does not get through.

While it may be possible that the child will get the message, will understand the seriousness, it is important to be sure this really is the case. Often these children will learn to say what the adults around them want to hear. For example, when asked "Do you want to be suspended?" or "Do you understand that this is a really big deal (or problem)?" the child will most certainly respond with what the adult wants to hear. They may have enjoyed their suspension or maybe they enjoy the excitement and attention or change. School policy can undermine progress in helping these children. If you are dealing with this issue, it is recommended you discuss this with a skilled advocate for guidance. You may also consider seeking information online via articles, forums or similar books like the one you are reading.

The most important thing is to remember that this is about the child. Try to understand their view, their world. Possibly they had a bad morning bus ride and it came out at 1pm as aggressive behavior. Maybe the child is frustrated they are unable to do certain work. There are so many factors here, so may points to work on and address. Try to stay calm, objective and constructive and help your child.

## ASPERGERS SCHOOL TUTORING

Do you think Aspergers school tutoring is an easy task? If you think so, you will need to know a lot about Aspergers syndrome. This syndrome is a mental illness. The patient suffers from deep depressions. The problem is very closely related to Autism. The students suffering from Autism or Aspergers syndrome are usually difficult to handle as their learning speed is very different from those of the kids who have a healthy mind. Aspergers syndrome is a mental illness which can make a healthy kid into a disabled one. The disability in case of Aspergers syndrome is not physical. It is mental disability. The student is simply not able to take care of him or herself. His or her mind is not as sharp as his or her school fellows. To keep themselves up to the mark, they need to work really hard. Aspergers syndrome is a difficult thing to handle and thus Aspergers school teaching can be taken as a challenge.

Aspergers school teaching deals with teaching the kids suffering from Aspergers. Kids suffering from Aspergers are not very bright. Aspergers school tutoring is thus not a very easy job. You need to have a lot of patience to conduct a class with the students suffering from autism or Aspergers syndrome. These kids are mentally disturbed ad thus it is very difficult for them to learn quickly. Aspergers school tutoring is thus a tough job for the teachers. Aspergers School tutoring in fact is a very difficult job. It requires a lot of patience. The teaching in this case does not only require your teaching skills but also your patience. Along with that, the teachers of these kids use a lot of strategies which make it easier for them to teach these kids with this mental disability. This disability may cause serious effects and the student may be disabled for the life. To avoid such situations it is important that teachers pay full attention towards Aspergers school teaching.

# CHAPTER FIFTEEN
# ASPERGER SYNDROME
# AND ANTIPSYCHOTICS

In recent years, psychiatrists have experimented with different kinds of medication for treating some of the negative effects of Asperger Syndrome, like irritability, depression, and hyperactivity. Unfortunately, a medication specifically targeted toward those with this condition is yet to be developed. However, researchers have found that many medications normally prescribed for disorders like schizophrenia are also safe to use in treating effects associated with Asperger Syndrome.

One such medication is Aripiprazole, more commonly known as Abilify. Abilify is an antipsychotic that was first developed to treat schizophrenia, but in November 2009, the FDA approved Abilify to be used by children ages 6 to 17 with Asperger Syndrome and other autism spectrum disorders. Studies have shown that it is also effective in treating irritability in adults, and there are many on the spectrum who take the drug.

Abilify was approved for treating depression in adults, which not only means that it can be prescribed to anyone on the spectrum who may see benefit from it, but depression is also another common effect of any Autism Spectrum Disorder. Abilify has the unique ability to help reduce irritability and meltdown severity while also helping to treat one of the most common co-morbid disorders that accompany Asperger Syndrome.

Abilify works by blocking receptors in the brain's dopamine pathways, which reduces the overall levels of dopamine in the brain. It is theorized that many mental disorders like schizophrenia and autism may be due to high levels of dopamine.

The medication's most common side effects for both children and adults are weight gain and increased appetite. Adults may also feel restless or anxious, or develop diabetes. Children, on the other hand, may feel lethargic. There are some more worrisome and even potentially permanent or fatal side effects, however, and a psychiatrist should always work to ensure that the potential benefits outweigh the risks, as well as monitor the patient for side effects.

Antipsychotics have caused some controversy in the past due to suicide attempts and suicidal thoughts associated with them. However, such extreme side effects are very rare. In fact, Abilify is classified as an atypical, or second-generation, antipsychotic, meaning that it is generally safer and more effective than traditional antipsychotics like Thorazine.

Abilify is most often taken as a pill, though it can also be injected. Finding the right dosage is a trial-and-error process. Psychiatrists will often under-prescribe patients at first, and then bump them up only if need be. It can take the body some time to adjust to the medication and respond. That's why it is important to not stop taking it, despite feeling better or like its no longer necessary.

Treating depression and decreasing irritability and meltdown severity have been two major challenges of treating Asperger Syndrome. That's why Abilify has been a great boon to the autism community.

COMMON DIAGNOSES COMORBID WITH ASPERGER SYNDROME

Many people today feel like they know a fair amount about Asperger Syndrome. They think the condition begins and ends with difficulty socializing and obsessive, highly specific interests. But that is only two of the many, many symptoms that characterize the condition. Asperger Syndrome can actually be very hard to diagnose, and in fact it is often mistaken as another mental disorder.

It's not that these other diagnoses are incorrect. Usually they are, in fact, present. It's just that they arise from the difficulties and symptoms of Asperger Syndrome. In other words, they are comorbid with autism-they are entirely separate conditions that accompany the primary diagnosis.

Here are the 3 most common comorbid conditions:

Anxiety Disorders

Social anxiety, obsessive-compulsive disorder, and generalized anxiety are all very common in those with Asperger

Syndrome. Some studies report that up to 84% of children with the condition also have some form of anxiety. Insecurity in their ability to interact with others, fear from departing from their routine, and other anxious feelings stem from its core symptoms.

Depression

Depression is a major problem in those with an Autism Spectrum Disorder. Some believe that their brain chemistry make them particularly susceptible, while others point out that isolation from peers, not being understood by others, and feelings of being "different" are all-too common and simple reasons that could led to depression.

Epilepsy/Seizures

It's reported that as many as one in four of those with some form of autism experience seizures. They're caused by abnormal electrical activity in the brain, and epilepsy comes from a frequent change in brain electrical activity. The link between the two has not been extensively studied, though it might point toward how autism affects the brain.

Comorbid conditions are often treated alongside Asperger Syndrome with little interruption in either treatment. In fact, many forms of therapy and medication can treat both at once. Abilify, for example, has been shown to alleviate depression and the irritability that arises in those with Asperger Syndrome.

Those who study and diagnose autism should always be aware of the many different ways it manifests and what separates it from other conditions. Studying its comorbidity can shed light on the condition itself and help further refine diagnostic tools. In this way, we can assure that people are seeking the correct treatment and getting the proper help they need.

## ASPERGER SYNDROME TEENAGERS AND VIOLENT BEHAVIOR, REBELLIOUS BEHAVIOR AND AGGRESSION

When it comes to Asperger Syndrome Behavior and teenager problems the teen years are the hardest. That is to say that the teen years are the hardest whether your child has Asperger's Syndrome or not! Raging hormones and frustration with social interactions at school can cause a lot of anger and bad behavior during the teen years.

Asperger Syndrome Behavior - Your child may have the need to:

Avoid responsibility - Attending school, obeying parents

Get something - His way in a decision, your attention, control over a situation

Manage pain - Physical and/or emotional

stress that must be alleviated

Fulfill sensory needs - Relief from heat, cold, or to satisfy thirstreb

Your child is unlikely to identify with your feelings or comprehend others' objections to his behavior. The only explanation you should use with him is to specifically state that the objectionable behavior is not permitted. Your son needs to follow rules, and following rules can help to focus and modify his rebellious behavior.

Asperger Syndrome Behavior modification

Behavior modification is a therapeutic approach that can change your son's behavior. You need to determine the need that his rebellion/aggression fulfils and teach him an acceptable replacement behavior. For example, your son can be taught to ask for, point to, or show an emotion card to indicate the need that he is trying to fulfill.

Asperger's Self-stimulating behaviors

Sometimes, self-stimulating behaviors such as rocking or pacing are taught as replacement behaviors, but it will take time for your son to integrate these behaviors into his daily activities. If your son is severely out of control, he needs to be physically removed from the situation. Granted, this may be easier said than done, and you may need someone to help you; yet, behavior modification can be helpful, and it must be started as soon as possible.

Maintaining a daily routine

For children and adolescents with Asperger's Syndrome, the importance of maintaining a daily routine cannot be stressed enough. A daily routine produces behavioral stability and psychological comfort for Asperger's children. Also, it lessens their need to make demands.

When you establish a daily routine, you eliminate some of the situations in which your son's behavior becomes demanding. For example, by building in regular times to give him attention, he may have less need to show aggression to try to get that attention.

Learn to recognize and communicate the causes of his aggression with your child

Ideally over time, your child will learn to recognize and communicate the causes of his aggression and get his needs met by using communication. Unfortunately, children who get their needs met due to aggression or violence are very likely to continue and escalate this oppositional behavior.

# COPING WITH ASPERGERS SYNDROME

## FACTORS TO SAFEGUARD YOUR CHILD'S WELFARE

Asperger's syndrome can constitute a challenging, and at times lonesome disorder for both children and their parents. Inherent in the disorders nature are difficulties associated with socializing and communicating with your toddler. Problems children have with peer communication and associated social behavior can also entail less play dates and birthday invitations. It can result in additional and frequently unwanted public scrutiny from those who simply do not understand that a child's meltdown constitutes part of impairment, and is not the consequence of "defective parenting."

Fortuitously, as Aspergers syndrome acquires widespread identification and attention, sources of assistance for parents of sufferers are becoming more prolific.

The following comprises some suggestions as to how to start actively coping with Aspergers in your family:

Ac uire knowledge about the disorder. As a stark comparison to even a decade ago, many pediatricians are well versed with Asperger's syndrome and the elements pertaining to a positive diagnosis. In addition, there are numerous books and internet sites committed to the disorder. Take the time to undertake the research so as to better understand the challenges being faced by your child, and the variety of services in your school district and community that may provide respite and assistance.

Learn to understand your child. The symptoms of Asperger's syndrome may follow a broad pattern but will be different for every child, and often depending on the circumstances in which the child finds themselves.

Often your child may struggle to verbalize their struggle, or fully comprehend much less rationalize the reasons for their behavior. However, with time and perseverance, you will be able to interpret which situations and environmental triggers are causing difficulties for your child. This in turn will assist in establishing and which coping strategies work. Consider the use of a diary to elucidate patterns in behavior or recurring problems.

Aᵭuaint yourself with relevant local professionals. Their advice will be integral in making key decisions in relation to your child's welfare, treatment and education. Use the advice available from those professionals and where possible, school counselors and teachers, to evaluate the options you have to develop a regime which can be most beneficial to your child. Contact social services and ask to have explained the federal regulations and potential benefits concerning children with impairments.

As many children have no overt signs of a disability, you will need to pro-actively advise and at times educate other family members, parents, and other adults involved with your child as to your child's special needs. This can avoid situations which may arise by virtue of a misunderstanding or miscommunication, which can nevertheless promote anxiety in your child, and otherwise exacerbate the difficulties your child may already be experiencing.

Assist your child in the challenge of creating passion from obsession. A typical behavior symptomatic of Aspergers disorder is the tendency to become fixated on a topic of narrow scope. This can prove frustrating and at times distracting to those upon whom your child's incessant discussion is influcted. However, an intense focus can also invigorate a child's connection to their education or social network. Frequently, this focus can enable a child to form lifelong pursuits of activities which permit them to actively contribute to their peer group, which in turn can ameliorate the isolation freЯuently experienced by individuals with Asbergers, and associated feelings of depression.

## IS ASPERGER SYNDROME SIMILAR TO AUTISM?

Asperger syndrome is a pervasive developmental disorder listed amongst those of the autism spectrum disorders. It is often closely compared with high functioning autism and some arguments dictate that it should be negated altogether and simply classified with high functioning autism. This syndrome is classified by a pattern of symptoms instead of just one symptom, such as impairment in social interaction, restricted patterns of behavior, activities and interests, there is no delay really in cognitive development however a significant delay in language is present. Those diagnosed with Asperger display an intense preoccupation or interest with particular subjects. They display a habit of excessive language defined as one-sided. They however also display a tendency towards restricted rhythms in their speech patterns. Sometimes those with Asperger can be physically clumsy and prone to accidents.

Life with this syndrome can be difficult but not impossible. In fact, there are those of a certain mind that consider any form of disorder from the autism spectrum to be a difference, not a disability. These of this persuasion advocate the necessity of treating such people as having mere differences, believing that both sides should simply take steps at accepting the other and working towards an easy cohabitation. Children born with this disorder or any other of this nature are not sick. They were born and began developing differences in their neural make up. Their brains began developing at a different rate as their bodies progressed steadily at the norm. These children are faced with altered factors in life, but this in no way makes them negatively different. Yes, children with Asperger and other such disorders will develop differently from other children. They will learn things differently, see things differently, and react to outside stimuli in a different manner. Still, these children, while living with a neuro-developmental disorder should not be considered a stigma.

It is important for any parent or caregiver of an Asperger child to know that these feelings of anxiety, fear, depression and anger towards the unfairness of it, are normal and that a diagnosis of Asperger is in no way a reflection on the parent(s) themselves. To help matters there are a variety of support groups and educational materials available to the public regarding this disorder and those like can look it up. Finding someone to talk to, a therapist, close friend, or the parent of another Asperger child is essential and can help with piece of mind. In fact, finding a support group made of parents for children with developmental disorders such as this can be beneficial to the parent and the child, as well as the siblings.

While there is no cure so to speak for Asperger syndrome, there are therapies that can be administered to alleviate the major difficulties a child will have functioning in normal life. Integrating them into a learning situation with others like then will help. And working at compromise throughout their daily schedules can be of great importance. It can be stressful for caregivers at times, but it is stressful for those with Asperger as well. Patience and a nurturing attitude will help all around.

# THE DIFFERENCE BETWEEN AUTISM AND ASPERGER SYNDROME

## Autism

Sometimes referred to as ASD, autism spectrum disorder is the general term used to identify a group of brain development disorders. Symptoms vary widely, though usually include problems with social interaction and both verbal and nonverbal communication. Other hallmarks of the condition are repetitive behaviors such as twirling or hand waving. Most children develop normally from birth and show signs of digression after the ages of one and two, losing language and social skills they started to develop.

Other signs are difficulty with social interactions, lack of eye contact, a hyper sensitivity to light, sound or the texture of foods and clothing. Slow language development or complete lack of, odd attachment to objects and a severe need to stick to rigid routines are also all signs. Those diagnosed often display increased or decreased reaction to pain, reaction to normal sound levels and an overwhelming need to withdraw from physical contact.

Believed to be caused by abnormal brain chemistry and physiology, the exact cause has not been identified. Many factors combine to produce the disorder, heredity, diet, mercury exposure, vitamin and mineral deficiencies, and even vaccine sensitivity.

According to the CDC, the center for disease control and prevention, one in every 68 children has been diagnosed, and although there's been no link to ethnic, racial or socioeconomic group, it is five times more likely to occur in boys. It is not uncommon to show average to above average intelligence.

# THE DIFFERENCE BETWEEN AUTISM AND ASPERGER SYNDROME

Considered a spectrum disorder, autism spectrum symptoms experienced can fall anywhere along a broad range of disability. This can range from those needing constant care and supervision to people who grow up and live independently, with social friends, families, homes and careers.

People with Asperger's are considered to have a high functioning form of autism. They typically do not talk sooner than other children, though often develop large vocabularies early and can converse on complex topics. They've earned the nickname "little professors" because of their intense ability to focus, and are quite often very successful academically.

Asperger symptoms can be very subtle and hard to exact. According to the website Autismspeaks.org, people with the syndrome are awkward in a way that is not easily understood. Trouble with eye contact and modulating their voices is common. They may fixate on a single subject that they find fascinating and talk incessantly about it without realizing that other people are not as interested. Mostly they long for normalcy and healthy connections much like other people do, though they may lack the skills to sustain them.

## HOW AN ASPERGER SYNDROME COMMUNITY CAN AID YOUR PARENTING

Asperger syndrome affects many around the globe. However, the wide dispersal which is associated with the condition normally leave several the feeling of isolation as they try to raise their kids with the limited knowledge available in the medical community.

The internet has helped in expanding the possibility of communication in many areas and for the parental community it has created new possibilities to meet and greet with other people who are sharing your life experiences. For the parent who has presently embraced the life of solitude when it comes to raising their child, it would be sensible to seek an on-line parental community which focuses on the raising of children with Asperger syndrome.

When you're able to access the opportunity of a community forum, you'll be able to gain experience in relation to this condition without actually going through the experiences. In these kinds of communities most parents are creating the possibility to communicate with other people so as to understand their experiences while sharing experiences of their own. The lesson of learning from people is essential in these types of venues, as it provides you with a one of a kind insight into raising your kid, that may not have been possible by attempting to raise your kid on your own. With this huge amount of experience at your hands you would be able to improve your parenting abilities as you provide your Asperger syndrome kid with the experiences which would exponentially benefit them.

The opportunity for a parent to meet with people who are sharing similar situations to your own is more important than any kind of knowledge or experience. The ability of the internet has expanded the size of a local community to a national or even global level, providing you access to people you would not have been able to make on your own. This level of support is essential for an individual, not just to further educate themselves on the Asperger syndrome, but to even communicate their achievements and frustrations with others.

This venue aids a person cope with the difficulties they may discover in this situation and have an outlet to access in order to develop friends. From a psychological point of view, individuals who communicate regularly with other people have a healthier approach to life's bumps over an individual who chooses to remain lone, permitting frustrations to build internally.

In life there are many road blocks which add complications and when you are forced to face those frustrations on your own they could build in a negative manner. Working with others offers a person with the possibility to build friendships, build off the experience of others and get knowledge that will be difficult to come by on your own.

## ASPERGERS SYNDROME IS NOT CURED WHEN REACHING ADULTHOOD

It is an often made mistake to think that 'it will go away', or that the problems almost all will have disappeared, when someone with Aspergers Syndrome has become an adult. On the contrary, there is a whole generation (or two) who were diagnosed with Aspergers Syndrome when they had been adults for many years already.

Of course children with Aspergers can learn a lot of skills and get rid of many 'bad habits', so that they can function reasonably well in everyday life. At least on the outside that seems to be the case. Also intellectually they are doing quite well. That might bare the danger in it that they often will encounter (to) high expectations, in more than one area of life.

Often this will lead to a lot of misunderstanding of their odd behaviors or mannerisms.

In reality adult men who have a certain pattern of deviant behavior, such as: lack of empathy, not being able to concentrate on more than one thing, often not being able to keep a job for a longer period of time, having problems with social skills, will get the diagnosis of Aspergers Syndrome quite late in their adulthood.

That is mostly after many years of problems and a lot of grieve for their partners and children, who will sometimes feel unloved or inadequate, and above all for themselves. They notice that they cannot function well in the society, often have all kinds of problems. They will be living with these questions on their minds: "Why do I fail so often in what I do? Why can I not do things that other people do so easily? Why do I have so little social contacts?" They may even think: "Am I crazy, or am I so very stupid?"

Then they might come to a certain point, for instance when the partner is totally at the end of her or his patience and understanding and threatens to leave, that the Aspergers will seek help. Mostly the first one they will turn to will be their G.P., who will probably refer them to a psychologist or some other specialist. If then, after years of struggling, it becomes clear what the matter is with this person, and if they will get help to learn how to cope with his or her Aspergers, then the pieces of the puzzle will finally fall into place, and they will be able to live a life with the Aspergers Syndrome.

Often, but not always, the relationship between the partners can be saved then, be it with different expectations. Having a father (or mother) or significant other with Aspergers Syndrome never will be easy, but sometimes worth the efforts, because Aspergers can be very good people to!

Still it can be very worthwhile to 'go the extra mile' for a (kind of) relationship with a person with Aspergers, because they often are good, interesting and intelligent people.

# CHAPTER SIXTEEN
# HOW TO ADVOCATE FOR YOUR CHILD WITH ASPERGER SYNDROME?

If your child was recently diagnosed with Asperger Syndrome, you will need to educate yourself about AS in order to understand how it affects him/her so that you can provide relevant information about his/her needs to the school in writing. You want to give the teacher as much information about your child as possible, in terms of how AS affects him/her, but at the same time keep the document as short as possible. That way the teacher is more likely to read ALL of it.

Here are a few points to consider including in your document:

Highlight the safety needs, both for your child and others. This will be the best way to get support for your child in the classroom (if that's what you want).

Think in terms of anxiety related behaviors and meltdowns that may lead to destructive behavior or aggressive behavior towards others, and the potential for your son or daughter to be the target of bullies.

Point out that although your son or daughter may look normal and advanced in many ways, he/she has poor communication skills because it is difficult for him/her to read facial expressions and make eye contact (if this is the case). Also he/she may take expressions literally and miss implied meanings. He/she may also have obsessive and limited interests and/or repetitive routines and physical clumsiness. Provide real examples that relate to your child. Remind the school that your child's ability to function well in group activities or social situations should not be over-estimated. As a result, he/she will need support and programming in all of these areas. Make suggestions as to what you would like to see in the IEP (Individual

Education Plan).

The teacher's attitude will be the prime example to a class on how to treat a child with Asperger Syndrome. If a teacher is intolerant and impatient with an AS student's odd behaviors, it sends a signal to the other students that it's okay to tease the AS student, both in and out of class. Also, it is important to point out that punishment is not the appropriate method for addressing the inappropriate behaviors of an AS student since the behaviors are one of the diagnostic signs and a result of having Asperger Syndrome.

You may want to consider disclosing the fact that your child has AS to the class. In my experience, other children are more likely to be tolerant of a student who acts and speaks in an odd way, if they know the reason.

If you decide to do this, here's a good tip. Write "Asperger Syndrome" on the board and stress the correct pronunciation to the class. This makes it less likely that the 'class clown' (every class has one) will hear the name as "Ass Burger" and make fun of your child using that term.

Your school may have anti-bullying policies in place which are not helping on a practical level. If your child is left unsupervised, he/she may become a victim of bullying but he/she may not have the skills to tell an adult. If you know or suspect that bullying is an issue, and the school or school board is unable or unwilling to deal with it appropriately, home schooling may be an option worth considering, even if only temporarily, since bullying will undoubtedly affect your child's emotional well-being.

# IMPORTANT ITEMS TO HELP YOU ADVOCATE FOR YOUR CHILD WITH ASPERGERS SYNDROME

Has your child recently been diagnosed with Aspergers Syndrome, and you are struggling to get your school district to recognize the diagnosis? Would you like to learn some important information to help you in your special education advocacy efforts, for your child? This article will specifically address things that you need to know to help you fight for special education services for your child.

Things that you need to know.

1. Aspergers Syndrome has its own category in the Diagnostic Statistical Manual (DSM IV) that is used for diagnosis. It is under the umbrella of Pervasive Developmental Disorders (PDD).

2. The American Psychiatric Association is proposing changing Aspergers Syndrome

from its own category to within the autism category for the DSM V. The intent is to try and make the diagnosis of autism clearer. The decision will be made within several months.

3. From an educational standpoint this is a wonderful decision, in my opinion, that will benefit thousands of children throughout the United States. Why? Many school districts have denied children with this disorder special education services because they state that the child does not have autism, and so therefore is not eligible. But in reality the Individuals with Disabilities Education Act state that a child must have one of 13 covered disabilities and have educational need. Aspergers is a part of the autism spectrum and should be a covered disability; though you may need to advocate for this.

4. Many children with this disorder will require help learning appropriate social

interactions and social skills. This should be provided as a special education services for your child if they need it. It could be working directly with a school social worker or participating in a small group social skills class.

5. Small groups may help your child with their education and also to develop appropriate social skills.

6. Modifications and adaptations in the regular classroom may help your child keep up with their peers.

7. Sensory integration disorder is common in many children with this disorder, and shows itself in difficulty with lights, sounds, different foods and different fabrics. If your child shows this difficulty, ask your school district for testing by an Occupational Therapist who is SIPT qualified (has received specialized training in the area of sensory integration/processing disorder).

8. Many children with Aspergers may need Occupational Therapy also for motor clumsiness. Ask for specific testing in this area if your child shows need.

ASPERGER SYNDROME QUESTIONS TO HELP TEACHERS

To help our kids who have Autism or Asperger Syndrome thrive in mainstream settings, you have to first pay attention to who they are as unique individuals.

Following are five key questions to help you reflect on what you are doing now and guide you to help these kids and adults have success:

1. Are you sure your child or student knows what it is you want him to do? Be sure the task is achievable and then be sure to understand the particular way he or she learns and acts on information. For example figures of speech are likely to confuse him,

while a visual demonstration or picture instructions are more likely to help him understand the task.

2. Do you have a plan or are you trying whatever technique comes to you as issues arise? Those effective techniues you use with your mainstream kids will probably let you down. You must have a program that orients around the needs and interests of your child or student with Autism or Asperger Syndrome. You have to really 'know your customer'. Spending time with a parent, last year's teacher or an IEP [Individualized Education Plan] to create a personalized behavior program will be well worth the time.

3. Are you focusing on past behaviors? Forget talking about what you don't want. Instead, teach specific new behaviors that replace inappropriate or unproductive behaviors. Take time to learn the strategies that will move your child forward and help

him grow independence. The more you practice new behavior skills, the more the wanted behaviors will grow and squeeze out the unwanted.

4. Are you feeding the potential for frenzy or working toward calm? Be aware of triggers and how you may be unintentionally setting them off all day long. Bright light, an odd smell in the room, discomfort when touched or bumped are the kinds of sensitivities you find with individuals on the autism spectrum. Try to accommodate their preferences and it is likely to pay off in better productivity.

5. Are you relying on punishment? Punishment invites crisis. Consequences invite problem solving. Consequences are the natural teachers. If you isolate your student with Asperger Syndrome for dominating the conversation in a class group, you are punishing, with no lesson to take from it. And your child will be further

confused. If you take the child aside, for a few minutes and some in-the-moment instruction about how to succeed at the group table, you are teaching necessary social skills and the way to avoid isolation in the future.

## STRATEGIES FOR TEACHING STUDENTS WITH ASPERGERS SYNDROME

It is not always very easy to teach students. There are students in a class who are bright and who are good at what they do. But it is a very frequent experiences of a teacher that there are students who are simply not interested in their work and they give a damn to whatever the teachers try to teach them. Sometimes you can blame the kid for this and sometimes you cannot. There are students who suffer from mental illness like Aspergers syndrome and it is seriously difficult for kids like that to focus on their students.

Strategies for teaching students with Aspergers syndrome are different than teaching ordinary healthy mind kids. The kids who have a healthy and bright mind could be taught very easily with the normal methods of teaching. Strategies for teaching students with Aspergers syndrome are different. The kids suffering from this syndrome have a different pace of learning and it is the responsibility of the teacher to understand their need and to focus on their requirements and teach them accordingly.

Strategies for teaching students with Aspergers syndrome are many but the best thing you need to do is to be patient. It is very difficult for the students who have this syndrome to work at the pace the students with healthy mind do. This increases the frustration of the kid suffering from autism or Aspergers syndrome. To avoid worse situations it is better that such kids are placed in a group which has as mix of students.

The kid needs to be appreciated again and again. His or her depression needs to be elevated. Once the depression is elevated, he or she will be able to work normally. But in the beginning the most important strategy a teacher should follow is that he or she needs to be patient with the kids.

Strategies for teaching students with Aspergers syndrome are different. It basically depends on the choice of the teachers as well as that of the students. The teachers understand their students in a better way and thus keeping this in mind, they work hard towards helping their student suffering from Aspergers syndrome to learn. This may be a slow process but teachers are made to fight with such situations.

## HOW TO USE YOUR DIAGNOSIS OF ASPERGER SYNDROME AS EMPOWERMENT

Living with Asperger Syndrome is an everyday challenge that makes every living moment a waking nightmare! But all of that will change if you just hang in there, take a moment every now and then to breathe, close your eyes, and just relax. When you found out that you were an Aspie, what went through your own mind? You probably zoned-out for a second, because you realized that you are not crazy or weird after-all!

Now that your diagnoses is out of the way, what about dealing with everyday issues? You may find that you are often misunderstood, that people just don't understand you, people who probably don't even want to understand you. How do you deal with that? Most of the time just telling them that you have Aspergers will only fall on deaf-ears.

I know, it's hard, but sometimes it is better to help other people understand your limitations, rather than just hiding behind your diagnoses.

When people understand your issues, they will more than likely try to adjust to better suit your needs. Don't fret if they forget, just give them a friendly-reminder. It's hard for anybody to be completely aware at all times of the day, so sometimes others will forget your limitations, they might forget that you aren't trying to be rude or anti-social, or they might think that you understand what they are trying to tell you when it isn't appropriate to assume so. They might think that you are being inappropriate. It takes some time to get used to the changes necessary.

You should understand that you can do anything that you want; you can be anything and anybody that you set out to be! Just realize that you have a unique perspective on life, and that those with Aspergers tend to have higher IQ-scores, so that means you generally have a higher-functioning brain than most people! Your brain is hard-wired for constant change, so use that to your advantage! Discuss your ideas and innovations with the world, and you may even inspire the greatest minds, and maybe you will change the minds of the more stubborn people! You can be very convincing.

The final thing you need to remember is that you are still a human-being, whether you are high-functioning or not, so don't see yourself as less-important, or someone that is unnatural! Your life matters, so help other people realize that!

## ASPERGER SYNDROME AND SENSORY OVERLOAD

## A MUM STORY

When my son had reached the age of 3 he was nearly impossible to handle. He would never go outside, refused to play with toys or go with me into the playground to play with the equipment there. He was scared when he was lifted off the ground and was terrified of swings and other equipment that would move. He was the only kid on the block who would never go on a kiddy-ride. He was unable to take a shower because he could not stand the water in his face, let alone go to the pool and swim! He was unable to get his hands dirty so playing with water and sand was impossible. He refused to put on new clothes due to the tags inside and was not able to eat solid food until the age of 3 and a half. I thought all three year old were this difficult to handle!

Apart from him being inside the house all day I was inside the house all day too. I was not allowed to sing, hum or whistle let along turn on a radio. He could not stand bright light or loud noises so he walked around all day with his ears covered with his hands. Even a simple thing as flushing the toilet was impossible due to the loud sound the water produces. I was unable to go out with him or visit friends with other kids. They were too loud. He would faint when the crowd on a birthday party would burst out in singing Happy Birthday.

For him this noise came out of the blue. A visit to the supermarket was a disaster due to all the loud noises and background music. On top of that he fainted about 6 times a day due to sensory overload. His nails and lips would go blue and he stopped breathing in, just out until his body went into complete shutdown. He started this when he was a 3 month old baby. We are not talking about kids with breath holding spell who will faint whenever they don't get their way or want more candy. This was different and it was obvious to us it was related to sensory issues.

For us help started in the form of an ORT who visited us at home. She had specialized in Sensory Integration Therapy and explained me all about it. Since we felt we had nothing to lose we started right away. It turned out the best thing that had happened to all of us! Even though the therapy is relatively easy to do and so much fun to participate in with your child, the results I have seen in my son were amazing. His therapy involved brushing, joint compression and sensory stimulation which have led to him calming down, being able to relax, eat solid foods and communicate with us in a much better way. He had so much fun doing it and it was never boring. After an initial 4 months of therapy at home he was able to go over to the practice of the ORT.

She had a huge swing set up for him, tunnels to crawl in, lost of soft materials to play with, music and all other fun stuff to keep my active toddler entertained. The results were amazing:

He started using different kinds of words and more words than ever before, we could go out, visit other families and go to the playground. The first time he asked if he could go on a kiddy ride I cried. He took swimming classes and now goes to the pool once a week. But the best reward of all is: he has not fainted anymore from the day the therapy started. I strongly believe all kids with oversensitive senses can benefit from this therapy, especially those with autism.

## CATCHING ASPERGER'S SYNDROME EARLY

Asperger's Syndrome is a problem with the brain that falls under the classification of

PDD (Pervasive Developmental Disorder). A child who is suffering with Aspergers Syndrome will have trouble socially and not have much interest in activities. When an activity is found that interests a child they will likely find comfort in repeating it, over and over.

Asperger's is similar to Autism. The main differences are that children with Asperger's have average to above average intelligence and are not impaired when it comes to language or helping themselves. They are likely to have a good vocabulary and speak the language just fine except that their speech will be in monotone.

Kids who have Asperger's Syndrome may or may not be antisocial. Learning the socialization skills that we take for granted, is never easy for them. They end up having extreme difficulty making friends and getting along with peers.

Boys are much more likely to get Asperger's Syndrome than girls. There has been no cure found for this condition. It is a lifelong condition. If a good treatment plan is followed the quality of life will be much better. It is possible to live a normal work life especially if the job does not require people skills.

The cause of Asperger's is related to bad genes that run in families. Problems in the family or being a bad parent does not contribute to this syndrome. Before Asperger's shows up there are often 'triggers' that show up out of nowhere. A sudden intolerance to certain foods might show up or a digestive problem will suddenly appear out of nowhere.

Asperger's Syndrome can often be controlled with herbal medicines. Herbs that are often beneficial include: St. John's Wort, Chamomile, Melissa Officinalis or Passiflora.

Make sure you talk with your doctor or homeopath before starting a treatment regimine. The type of pill you give to your child might contain a certain combination of herbs in order to have the desired effect. The right kind of holistic treatment plan will aim to address the underlying problem instead of simply treating the symptoms.

If your child is diagnosed with Asperger's Syndrome make sure that you learn everything you can about it. Focusing on your child's strengths can really help them to excel in life. If they develop a strong interest in a particular subject then make sure you encourage them by providing reading and learning materials on that subject. Someday, they may even turn it into a career.

# THE ASPERGER'S LABEL - DOES IT STICK?

Labels can be tricky. They don't always stick.

As more and more of us have become familiarized with terms like "autism" and "Asperger Syndrome", many have begun to wonder if the increase in its occurrence is less a matter of an epidemic and more a matter of what is in vogue - after all, the label "Asperger's" is applied to people who display dramatically different symptoms, and there is little agreement about causes, and even treatment.

"Do you specialize in working with adults with Asperger's?" - This is a question I field many times a week individuals and couples calling seeking psychotherapy services. Though my answer is always "yes", there are many in the field who might argue that the answer should be "no". Some might assert that I, in fact, work only with adults who have "Asperger's like coping mechanisms".

Am I applying the Asperger's label too liberally? A debate has flared amongst clinicians, researchers and clients themselves regarding the official diagnosis of Asperger Syndrome. In one camp are those who adhere rigidly to diagnostic criteria listed in the DMS-IV (the profession's manual for diagnosing disorders). These professionals view the individual with "true Asperger's" as not only displaying difficulty in connecting with others, but lack of interest. "Almost by definition, an Asperger's person would not form an intimate relationship, get married and have children," says research scientist Katherine Tsatsanis of the Yale Developmental Disabilities Clinic. "They don't form connections. The desire, the drive and the social knowledge is lacking."

In the second camp are professionals who work with individuals who have lived lives largely feeling isolated, cerebral and confused by the nuances of interpersonal relationships? Some are married, some are not. Some love computers, some English. They are professors, pilots, graphic artists, forest rangers, electricians, bakers, computer scientists, physicians. Perhaps what they often have in common are characteristics not normally listed in the DSM-IV or surveyed with research scales: a love of and identification with cats, an intense sensitivity sometimes hidden by a shut-down or disengaged persona, an eschewing of group sports, a simultaneous craving for solitude and longing for companionship.

Which camp's perspective you subscribe to may depend on whether labeling works for you. The very nature of spectrum disorders can make diagnosing complex and difficult. If you have a questions about whether the label is right for you or someone you love, keep in mind that the more important question may be this: do you need a label?

For some, having a name for a set of experiences and characteristics which has caused pain and confusion throughout life can be a great relief. Having a name for "what's wrong" can feel organizing, provide a context for approaching treatment, de-mystify previously confusing parts of life, and depersonalize the pain that has come with being different. Naming can be a triumph in itself.

For others, labeling can cause distress, even worsen feelings of being different or flawed. For these folks, organizing and context are less valuable. If the diagnosis causes further pain, it may not be useful. Why? Because of the spectrum nature of Pervasive Developmental Disorders. Asperger's Syndrome is known by many names - High Functioning Autism (HFA), Autism Spectrum Disorder (ASD), and others. The term "spectrum" is crucial to the understanding of how these disorders present in terms of symptoms and severity.

To assume that all adults with the diagnosis display the same characteristics would be to miss the true nature of the disorder, which often forces individuals to develop widely varying and novel ways of coping with sensory input, social expectations and neurological wiring.

If you or a loved one suspect the Asperger's label may be applicable, you may want to consult with a professional for confirmation. Or not. Depending on how much you need to name what's different about you, you may want to skip this step and just address symptoms. And if you do walk out of a professional's office with the label "Asperger Syndrome", just remember that the label may not stick.

# ASPERGER GIRLS: THE PROBLEM WITH GENDER

Asperger Syndrome is an ever-more-common neurological condition. Under the autism umbrella, it is also one of the most complex and misunderstood.

However, no matter how many difficulties an "Aspie" (A self-coined nickname) may suffer, there is one that vexes many teen and adult Aspies. However, as it (in 98% of cases) affects mostly females with the condition - "Aspergirls" - so here we go.

In most cases, Aspergirls have a blurring line between their ideas of gender. While this may simply cause a case of simple tomboy activity, it has been known to commonly range from bisexuality to full-blown gender androgyny. Androgyny here meaning 'no preference between the genders, reflected in image, activities and belief.

Most parents may be worried or upset by their previously girly little angels becoming more and more gender-fluid by the day. However, most Aspergirls prefer to be in no gender stereotype. While they may gain negative attention due to their gender ambiguity, they are in fact more anxious when placed in a conforming gender stereotype.

Society is changing every day, and gender-fluidity is welcomed. Mechanics, engineering, there are many careers that can suit an Aspergirl, and where ambiguity is certainly welcomed!

Is your Aspergirl a slightly boyish character? Then embrace it! In the end, she is happy, and she will choose her own path. Support her and her image choices, and do not push her towards femininity or dating, long hair, makeup and girl activities.

## ASPERGERS SYMPTOMS & ASPERGERS DIAGNOSIS

As there are no specific genetic or biological markers indicative of a person being afflicted with Autism Spectrum Disorder, Aspergers diagnosis is as a matter of necessity based on behavior. The Autism Spectrum Disorder ("ASD") is used to describe a series of related disorders which can include Aspergers disease, autism, Pervasive Developmental Disorder Not Otherwise Specified ("PDD-NOS") and is often displayed in conjunction with ADHD.

For those looking to identify Aspergers symptoms as a precursor to Aspergers diagnosis, there are three main areas of difficulty which are common to people with Aspergers. These are:

1. Impairment in social interaction

2. Impairment in communication

3. Restricted and/or repetitive patterns of

behavior, interests and activities

Not all sufferers will display each Aspergers symptoms and the severity and presence of each symptom may vary. However, Aspergers typically manifests in childhood, with onset and diagnosis being possible from approximately 3 years and over.

Social Interaction Impairment

Whilst Aspergers symptoms can be varied, they fre□uently include marked difficulties with nonverbal behavior such as interpreting body language, eye contact, understanding or utilizing appropriate facial expression, and other cues commonly associated with regulating social expression. Fre□uently this type of Aspergers symptom will impact upon a person's capacity to form relationships within their peer group, and can be accompanied by an apparent lack of social empathy or an inability to see the perspectives of others. In children, this extends beyond age appropriate egocentricity.

## Difficulties with communication

Delayed development of linguistic abilities when accompanied with an inability to adopt an alternative strategy to communicate is one of the recognized Aspergers Symptoms. Whilst language development may appear normal, people with Aspergers will often utilize repetitive speech patterns, and be delivered with an absence of varying tone or pitch.

## Restricted behavior, interests & activities

When considering whether an Aspergers diagnosis may be needed, one of the symptoms to be aware of is when an intense interest in one specific type of activity is prevalent. Such interests may be diverse, but tend towards a focus on a part rather than a whole. For example, it may be a fascination with spinning a wheel on a toy truck, or a pre-occupation with something as seemingly mundane as a fan motor. What is significant is that the interest consumes an unusual quantity of time and focus.

Similarly, two other Aspergers Symptoms are inflexibility in changes in routine, and the associated distress with any such changes. When anxious, people with Aspergers disorder may be prone to repetitive mannerisms which are indicative of heightened stress levels, such as finger flicking or hand motions.

Other behavior symptomatic of Aspergers

In addition to the Asperger's syndrome symptoms above, many professionals will include other behavior as part of their Aspergers diagnostic criteria. A heightened response to sensory stimuli, latent gross motor skills, sleep disturbances and high pain tolerance are just some of the additional factors which may be attributable to a positive Aspergers diagnosis.

If you are concerned that a loved one or child may be suffering from Aspergers syndrome, there is a large body of information available to assist in taking the first positive steps towards diagnosis and management. Whilst the precise cause of Aspergers is not yet known, there are established methods of treatment, and early diagnosis of asperger's syndrome in children can be instrumental in minimizing the impact Aspergers may have on the sufferer.

# CONCLUSION

Aspergers Syndrome is a developmental disorder classified under "pervasive development disorder" (PDD). In lay terms, this means that individuals with Aspergers Syndrome have delays in the development of multiple basic functions, especially around socialization and communication. It is estimated that 1 in 277 of all children suffers from Aspergers Syndrome.

Aspergers Syndrome and Autism are different grades in a spectrum of developmental disorder. It is similar to classic Autism in a variety of ways but differs mainly because Aspergers Syndrome individuals are usually higher functioning. IQ tests may show superior intelligence or even a very high memory capacity in individuals diagnosed with Aspergers Syndrome. Some of the differences from Autism include:

Onset of symptoms is usually later in Aspergers Syndrome

Social and communication deficits are less severe in Aspergers Syndrome

Circumscribed interests are more prominent in Aspergers Syndrome

Verbal IQ is usually higher than performance IQ (in autism, the case is usually the reverse)

Family history is more frequently positive in Aspergers Syndrome

Due to lack of physical manifestations, and variability in presentation, Aspergers Syndrome is often not identified in early childhood; in fact, many individuals are not diagnosed until they are adults!! Although children with Aspergers Syndrome tend to look exactly like other children, they behave differently. These results in the following:

Siblings feel embarrassed around peers; often times frustrated by not having the relationship they expected with their sibling and most importantly feel angry because children with Aspergers Syndrome reuire a lot of parent's time.

Frustration for parents; Parenting a child with Aspergers Syndrome can be frustrating, tiring and demanding. It is hard enough for parents to understand why their beloved child has this disorder. It is even more difficult to understand and relate to the child behavior triggered by no "apparent" cause. Child with Aspergers Syndrome may start hitting family members, shout and scream without any apparent cause.

As a result of this parents and siblings can get overwhelmed in coping with the behavior arising as a result of Aspergers Syndrome. Other times it may even disrupt peace at home. This further worsens the

Childs behavior and hence a vicious circle ensues. Although children with Aspergers Syndrome tend to look exactly like other children, they behave differently.

These results in the following:

Siblings feel embarrassed around peers; often times frustrated by not having the relationship they expected with their sibling and most importantly feel angry because children with Aspergers Syndrome require a lot of parent's time.

Frustration for parents; Parenting a child with Aspergers Syndrome can be frustrating, tiring and demanding. It is hard enough for parents to understand why their beloved child has this disorder. It is even more difficult to understand and relate to the child behavior triggered by no "apparent" cause. Child with Aspergers

Syndrome may start hitting family members, shout and scream without any apparent cause.

As a result of this parents and siblings can get overwhelmed in coping with the behavior arising as a result of Aspergers Syndrome. Other times it may even disrupt peace at home. This further worsens the Childs behavior and hence a vicious circle ensues. Although there is no definitive "cure" Aspergers Syndrome, treatment is given around the core symptoms of:

Poor communication skills

Obsessive or repetitive routines

Physical clumsiness

A typical treatment program to Aspergers Syndrome generally includes; Social skill training; Cognitive behavior therapy; Medications, mainly for depression, anxiety, and ADD/ADHD; Occupational or physical therapy; Specialized speech therapy; Parent training and support

It is important that parents have a good understanding of what Aspergers Syndrome is? It is important for the child that siblings and family are explained about the syndrome (to help them deal with it better). Furthermore focused activities should be planned with the child everyday e.g. swimming, shopping, etc; Parents should attempt to make the child's childhood as "normal" as possible (It is tempting for the parents and siblings to cuddle the child with Aspergers Syndrome) - this is important so that the child can have similar childhood as their siblings e.g. sibling rivalry, fighting over toys, TV shows, etc. Dealing with a child with Aspergers Syndrome can get challenging. With some help and guidance, it can help the parents and the child a long way, in how to deal with day to day scenarios and to keep peace in their families.